I0767132

The **Little** 21
and Beyond
Lifestyle Journal

Tips on the Principles of Health and Wellness

DONETTE WYNTER

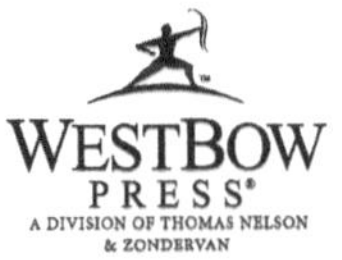

WESTBOW
PRESS®
A DIVISION OF THOMAS NELSON
& ZONDERVAN

WestBow Press books may be ordered through booksellers or by contacting:

WestBow Press
A Division of Thomas Nelson & Zondervan
1663 Liberty Drive
Bloomington, IN 47403
www.westbowpress.com
1 (866) 928-1240

ISBN: 978-1-9736-7711-6 (sc)
ISBN: 978-1-9736-7713-0 (hc)
ISBN: 978-1-9736-7712-3 (e)

Library of Congress Control Number: 2019915933

Print information available on the last page.

WestBow Press rev. date: 10/22/2019

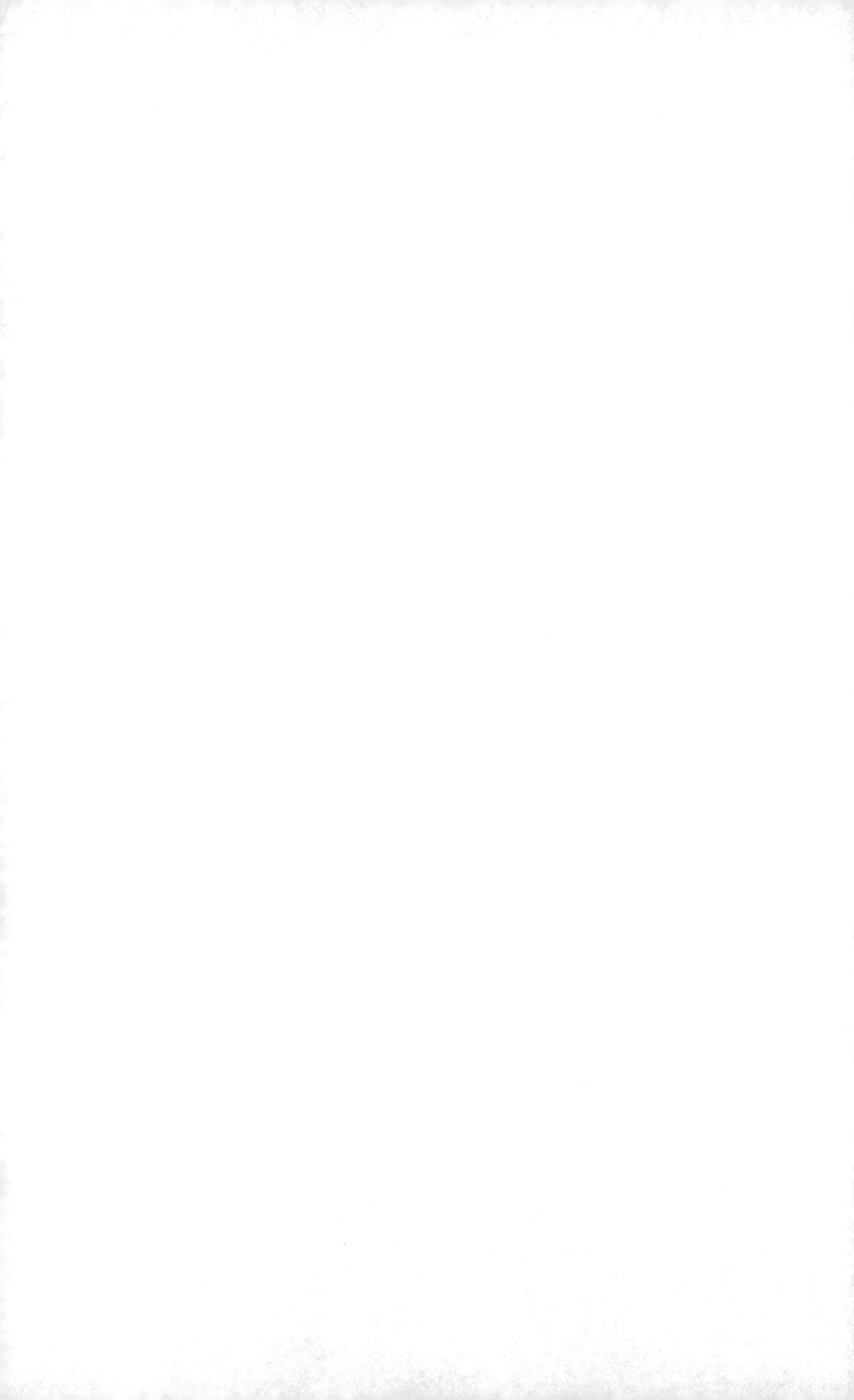

Introduction

Our health is the most valuable commodity we possess while on this journey of life. The World Health Organization defines health as, "a state of complete physical, mental and social well-being and not merely the absence of disease or infirmity." Implicit in that definition is the fact that health is multifaceted and cannot be considered without the careful integration of all component parts: mind, body and spirit. To achieve optimal health, there are pertinent questions to consider. What am I thinking? What is my belief system with regards to my mind, body and spirit? What are my coping strategies? How much exercise do I get? What are my dietary choices? What are the daily actions I engage in that negatively or positively affect my health? All the answers to those questions will be a good indicator of our daily health habits.

The daily practices we engage in will determine which end of the spectrum of wellness we find ourselves eventually as health is not static but moves up or down on a continuum. If it is the epitome of health or constantly battling something, it is dependent on the personal responsibility for our health that we assume. The quality of life or level wellness is all up to the individual. Wellness focuses on the complete person, (mind, body and spirit) not just on the physical.

It does not matter where you are on this continuum of wellness it can get better. As long as there is life there is hope. **WELCOME** to the first step of the rest of your most abundant life.

The little 21 and beyond Lifestyle journal is a useful tool that will facilitate the change process on your wellness journey. Dr Maxwell Maltz in the 1950's found that it took a minimum of about 21 days to form a new habit. With the use of this knowledge we lay this new foundation of health and wellness beginning with just 21 days.

This is a catalyst to creating the more complete you. All that is required is to make the decision for change, commit to the process and the rest is history. Before starting one is encouraged to make personal goals and write them on the page in the allotted spaces provided. Inside these pages are Tips on the principles of health, Space to write daily power thoughts to meditate on that will transform your minds, and the opportunity to chronicle your journey to the new, better, more empowered you.

Almost on a weekly basis somebody says to me it is expensive to eat right but I dare to challenge this thought. Where there is a will there is a way. Yes and we always say "we get what we pay for" we will buy the expensive shoe, the dream car etc. but how much are we willing to spend on our health. The wisest man said "Buy the truth, and do not sell it, also wisdom, and instruction, and understanding". As it is said "prevention is better than cure." Make the decision, take the steps and invest in the future. There is no better time than the present to turn over a new leaf. Our decisions and actions today are the seeds we sew and we will reap the harvest tomorrow once it matures. Then we would have a heritage to pass on to the next generation.

My commitment
I am destined for purpose and so
I pledge to make my health (mind, body and spirit) a priority
So that I can accomplish all that I was placed on this earth to do.

Your name

There is value in a Friend/partner
Get someone to take the journey with you,
There is strength in unity.

Principles of Health and Healing

Our body is an amazing self-healing system created for good works and is able to do just that once given the right condition in which to function. The human body is sacred, actually a "temple" and we should treat it as such. There are some basic principles of health and healing which are universal and do not change regardless of race, culture, climate etc. The principles of health and healing highlighted are as follows:

Belief: Any real and permanent change begins in the mind. Our beliefs shape our values, philosophies, source of motivation, our actions and ultimately our health status. What I am saying is that we can only be transformed when our minds are renewed. Our thought processes determine our reality so be very careful what you are thinking. Change your mind, change your heart, change your words, change your reality and change your destiny. You can do whatever we are able to make a picture of.

Words: The words we speak will create our reality. The spring of life resides in the tongue, and so we should not say anything we do not desire to manifest and become our truth. We can change our reality, by changing our thoughts, which will change our words. We can change our thoughts by meditating on new things.

Pure air: We live in a toxic world. The lung is one of the routes through which these toxins get into our bodies. Environmental pollutants are all around us and are unavoidable. They are actually most prolific in our homes, from the toxic fumes in the cleaning agents, to the carpet, paint, and furniture, air fresheners, perfumes, pesticides, plastics etc. Research has shown that the outside air is cleaner than the air in our homes. Our homes should be well ventilated with fresh oxygenated air flow. The practice of deep breathing of clean early morning mountain air is best. When you breathe in, your belly should expand. When you breathe out, your belly should fall.

Eliminate anything injurious: This involves being self controlled in our eating and drinking. As best as possible avoid anything that is potentially harmful like coffee, alcohol, foods that are high in sugars, fats, additives & preservatives including: Dairy products, large amounts of meat, pastries, chips and dips, sweets, refined breads, frozen dinners, and fast foods.

Sunlight: The body makes vitamin D when the skin is exposed to the ultraviolet B (UVB) rays in sunlight. About 5 to 30 minutes of exposure in the early morning (without sunscreen) is good. It is commonly said that excess sunlight causes cancer, however the absence of sunlight increases the risk of many cancers and osteoporosis, because of the absence of circulating Vitamin D-3 and its derivatives. Vitamin D plays a vital role in the immunity, blood cell formation and cancer fighting properties.

Rest: Sleep recharges our batteries. Sleeping in the dark is a key to health maintenance. Sleep prior to mid night is better than sleep after midnight. The goal should be eight hours per night. If we do so we will secrete a hormone Melatonin which is produced in the pineal gland. It regulates other hormones and the sleep cycle. It is the most powerful antioxidant and a free radical scavenger. It is an immune enhancer as it fights against inflammation. It peaks in our bodies between the hours of 2-3am while asleep in the dark after daytime exposure to sunlight. If the daytime sunlight is too little then the production goes down.

Exercise: One could easily say use it or lose it relation to the human body. The body is like a machine and exercise maintain the systems (respiratory, cardiovascular, digestive, neuro-muscular, lymphatic, etc. Without exercise ideal health would be a pipe dream. One must engage in about one hour of physical activity daily. You can begin with even 15 minutes and increase over time. Strength training exercise results in a leaner more agile body. This is one sure way to add years to our life and quality to the years.

Proper diet: This is one which includes living, plant based items, which was created as food and grown in an environment free from harmful substances. This should include at least 5-9 servings of fruits and vegetables daily with more vegetables than fruits. Have whole grain breads and cereals, at least 3 servings daily, including brown rice and oatmeal. Peas, beans, nuts, organic soy foods, hemp powder are good sources of plant protein. Good quality protein from animals allowed to free range is preferred if meat is included in the diet. Do not wait too long to eat and get very hungry; ideally have three square meals with a fruit or vegetable snack in between each meal. To avoid binge eating be sure to pack a lunch bag with wholesome snacks on a daily basis. Knowledge and use of herb will also be beneficial for health maintenance.

Eat slowly: Take small bites and completely chew food until it is a liquid, to aid in ease of digestion which really begins in the mouth. If we take note the persons around us who take a long time to eat their meals are often not overweight. The fullness of our stomach does not register right away in the brain so it is easy to overeat if we rush. The reason we rush is often the pressure to get to another activity. The body reads this as stress and the body's natural response to stress is to slow down or completely stop the digestion process. On more than one counts it is beneficial to eat slowly.

The use of water: Water makes up more than two-thirds of the weight of the human body. Without water, we will die. All the cells and organs need water to function. Distilled water is void of contamination. Water literally washes our cells, it is a lubricant, regulates body temperature, and the medium of transportation of water soluble nutrients to the cells and toxins from the cells.

Aromatherapy: This involves the sense of smell and the use of highly concentrated essential anointing oils distilled from plants such as myrtle, coriander, hyssop, galbanum, and rosemary for healing purposes. This just increases general wellbeing.

Use of Music: Music is known to lift the spirit. Incorporating classical music is beneficial in retraining the brain to relax. There are no claims to fame that music can cure cancer or any other diseases, but Health care professionals believe it can reduce some symptoms, aid in healing, improve overall physical rehabilitation, facilitating movement, and enrich quality of life.

Trust in Divine power: Prayer can provide us healing for our wounded hearts and mind, victory over much of life's challenges. If one is able to depend on someone greater than the self then the burdens of life becomes a lot easier to carry.

Be kind to self and others: Negative emotions whoever it is directed will produce the stress reaction in your body. Replace negative thoughts and emotions with positive ones. Do not judge yourself or others. Instead, love and accept yourself where you are and do the same for others.

Adequate Stress Management: We live in a highly stressful world. From morning till night we rush from one stressor to another. Walter Cannon of Harvard University first described the "Stress Response" and its link to the "fight or flight" hormone cortisol. The perceived stress sets up a cascade of events in our bodies. Continuous stress if not dealt with leads to burn out and potentially even death. It does pay to be anxious for nothing, and guard your heart. Make every effort to cultivate a gentle and quiet spirit. To counteract stress learn and implement strategies of daily relaxation.

Relaxation: Herbert Benson of Harvard Medical School described the "relaxation response". It is the opposite of the stress response and as such there are tremendous benefits to be derived from engaging our minds and changing the hormones circulating in our bodies and the outcome of our health. We cannot change the potentially stressful events in our lives but we can choose how we respond to them. There are basic, simple relaxation techniques that can be taught.

Fasting: This is the abstinence from all food. This can be beneficial when done for a short period of time as the body gets the opportunity to rest and repair.

Before Fasting: Visit your doctor to make sure it is safe to do so. Prepare body before a fast you must start 5-6 days prior to the fasting period and eliminate processed foods. About the third day take a mild laxative to help expel toxins from your body. This process lessens the side effects of fasting example headaches, nausea, vomiting, weakness etc.

Breaking the fast: Sweet fruits or their juices are used to break a fast, the common fruits: grapes, musk melon, water melon, pears, apples, oranges, pineapples, papayas, etc. Start by eating small portions chewing slowly to stimulate the production of saliva, gastric juices and intestinal movement. This should be done every hour or more if the stomach maintains a sensation of fullness or bloating with gas. During the days following you can take larger portions with longer intervals of time in between.

If you break the fast with juice, it must be fresh natural juice served at room temperature. This must be taken in small quantities slowly to avoid pains. The quantity can vary between ½ -1 glass every 1-2 hour respectively. On the following days the quantity can increase to longer time intervals.

The benefits of fasting are: promoting detoxification, resting the digestive system, resolving inflammatory responses, reducing blood sugar, increasing fat breakdown, correction of high blood pressure, promotion of weight loss, promoting a healthy diet, boosting immunity, and helping to overcome addictions.

Fasting for long periods of time is bad for you. Your body needs to be nourished on a daily basis with the richness we receive from bountiful harvest that the earth produces. Without the essential elements it is only a matter of time before our body complains. Fasting too long can be life-threatening.

Be Thankful: It does not matter how dim life is a thankful mind will see the world through beautiful lenses. The brain actually produces beneficial hormones which impacts positively on the body, so daily look for things to be thankful for.

Smile Often: A smile not only lifts the spirit of the person in front of you but it also lifts your own. I often say even a fake smile is better than a frown.

Purposeful Living: Do you rise in the morning with a sense of purpose, focused on a meaningful goal that you deliberately work at achieving, or do you wish you did not have to go to work or deal with that person today. STOP!!! Check your life. If you can't find joy in each new day, then start asking some quality questions like: Why am I still alive? What is that one thing that I need to accomplish with the rest of my life? Whose life do you have the power to impact positively? Then do it.

If the job or whatever is the reason you can't accomplish that one thing you always knew you needed to do, then start asking the questions; What else can I do to still earn, maybe less but I will have the time to accomplish that thing? What else can I do differently to make sure I accomplish that thing and start living with purpose?

There is a specific audience that only you can reach. Their lives depend on you walking in your purpose. If you don't walk in your purpose, they may never get to walk in their purpose. Not being aware of and living with purpose is like being alive but dead.

When the answers to the questions asked come to you, even if it is unpopular and looks ridiculous to others around you, do not rationalize them away and daily choose to live extraordinarily in all areas of life. Now own this process. Carefully craft some specific goals on the next page, using the guidelines provided.

Goal Setting: This is one of the most significant steps in the process of changing your lifestyle. We are encouraged to write a personal vision. It should have a greater good higher than ones' self. It should be what you want and not what anyone else wants. It should be achievable and sustainable. It should be positively stated (example: I will), measureable (example: lose 5 pounds) and time sensitive (example: in 21 days).

You have gotten this far. Congrats take the next step.

Date: / /

My goals

Mind ____
____

Body ____
____

Spirit ____
____

Relationships ____
____

Family ____
____

Business ____
____

School ____
____

Career ____
____

Generally ____
____
____
____
____
____
____
____
____
____
____
____
____
____
____

Day 1

Power thought/quote:____

What are you thankful for today? _______________________________
____
____

Quiet time 5-10 minutes: Listen, read, meditate, write daily goals

____
____
____

Exercise: choose any activity you enjoy that will increase your heart rate to a point where you can answer a question but not carry on a conversation. Average 30 minutes. ____

Breakfast: ____
Snack:____
lunch:____
Snack:____
Dinner: ____

Quiet time: Before bed take 15 minutes to reflect on the day. How did you do? Be kind and forgiving to self and others.

Mind ____
____
Body ____
____
Spirit ____
____
Relationships____
____
Family ____
____
Business____
____
School ____
____
Career ____
____

Day 2

Power thought/quote: ____

What are you thankful for today? _______________________________________

____

____

Quiet time 5-10 minutes: Listen, read, meditate, write daily goals

____

____

____

Exercise: choose any activity you enjoy that will increase your heart rate to a point where you can answer a question but not carry on a conversation. Average 30 minutes. ____

Breakfast: ____

Snack:____

lunch:____

Snack:____

Dinner: ____

Quiet time: Before bed take 15 minutes to reflect on the day. How did you do? Be kind and forgiving to self and others.

Mind ____

____

Body ____

____

Spirit ____

____

Relationships ____

____

Family ____

____

Business____

____

School ____

____

Career ____

____

Day 3

Power thought/quote: ____

What are you thankful for today? ____
____
____

Quiet time 5-10 minutes: Listen, read, meditate, write daily goals
____
____
____

Exercise: choose any activity you enjoy that will increase your heart rate to a point where you can answer a question but not carry on a conversation. Average 30 minutes. ____

Breakfast: ____
Snack:____
lunch:____
Snack:____
Dinner: ____

Quiet time: Before bed take 15 minutes to reflect on the day. How did you do? Be kind and forgiving to self and others.

Mind ____
____

Body____
____

Spirit ____
____

Relationships____
____

Family ____
____

Business____
____

School ____
____

Career ____
____

Day 4

Power thought/quote: ____

What are you thankful for today? ________________________________

____

____

Quiet time 5-10 minutes: Listen, read, meditate, write daily goals

____

____

____

Exercise: choose any activity you enjoy that will increase your heart rate to a point where you can answer a question but not carry on a conversation. Average 30 minutes. ____

Breakfast: ____

Snack:____

lunch:____

Snack:____

Dinner: ____

Quiet time: Before bed take 15 minutes to reflect on the day. How did you do? Be kind and forgiving to self and others.

Mind ____

____

Body ____

____

Spirit ____

____

Relationships ____

____

Family ____

____

Business____

____

School ____

____

Career ____

____

Day 5

Power thought/quote: ____

What are you thankful for today? ____________________________________
____
____

Quiet time 5-10 minutes: Listen, read, meditate, write daily goals
____
____
____

Exercise: choose any activity you enjoy that will increase your heart rate to a point where you can answer a question but not carry on a conversation. Average 30 minutes. ____

Breakfast: ____
Snack:____
lunch:____
Snack:____
Dinner: ____

Quiet time: Before bed take 15 minutes to reflect on the day. How did you do? Be kind and forgiving to self and others.

Mind ____
____

Body ____
____

Spirit ____
____

Relationships____
____

Family ____
____

Business____
____

School ____
____

Career ____
____

Day 6

Power thought/quote: ____

What are you thankful for today? ______________________________________

____

____

Quiet time 5-10 minutes: Listen, read, meditate, write daily goals

____

____

____

Exercise: choose any activity you enjoy that will increase your heart rate to a point where you can answer a question but not carry on a conversation. Average 30 minutes. ____

Breakfast: ____

Snack:____

lunch: ____

Snack:____

Dinner: ____

Quiet time: Before bed take 15 minutes to reflect on the day. How did you do? Be kind and forgiving to self and others.

Mind ____

____

Body ____

____

Spirit ____

____

Relationships____

____

Family ____

____

Business____

____

School ____

____

Career ____

____

Day 7

Power thought/quote: _______________________________________

What are you thankful for today? _______________________________

____

____

Quiet time 5-10 minutes: Listen, read, meditate, write daily goals

____

____

____

Exercise: choose any activity you enjoy that will increase your heart rate to a point where you can answer a question but not carry on a conversation. Average 30 minutes. ____

Breakfast: ____
Snack:____
lunch: ____
Snack:____
Dinner: ____

Quiet time: Before bed take 15 minutes to reflect on the day. How did you do? Be kind and forgiving to self and others.

Mind ____

____

Body ____

____

Spirit ____

____

Relationships____

____

Family ____

____

Business____

____

School ____

____

Career ____

____

Day 8

Power thought/quote: _______________________________________

What are you thankful for today? _______________________________

____

____

Quiet time 5-10 minutes: Listen, read, meditate, write daily goals

____

____

____

Exercise: choose any activity you enjoy that will increase your heart rate to a point where you can answer a question but not carry on a conversation. Average 30 minutes. _______________________________________

Breakfast: ____
Snack:____
lunch:____
Snack:____
Dinner: ____

Quiet time: Before bed take 15 minutes to reflect on the day. How did you do? Be kind and forgiving to self and others.

Mind ____

____

Body ____

____

Spirit ____

____

Relationships____

____

Family ____

____

Business____

____

School ____

____

Career ____

____

Day 9

Power thought/quote: ____

What are you thankful for today? _______________________________________

____

____

Quiet time 5-10 minutes: Listen, read, meditate, write daily goals

____

____

____

Exercise: choose any activity you enjoy that will increase your heart rate to a point where you can answer a question but not carry on a conversation. Average 30 minutes. ____

Breakfast: ____

Snack:____

lunch:____

Snack:____

Dinner: ____

Quiet time: Before bed take 15 minutes to reflect on the day. How did you do? Be kind and forgiving to self and others.

Mind ____

____

Body ____

____

Spirit ____

____

Relationships____

____

Family ____

____

Business____

____

School ____

____

Career ____

____

Day 10

Power thought/quote: _______________________________________

What are you thankful for today? _______________________________
____
____

Quiet time 5-10 minutes: Listen, read, meditate, write daily goals

____
____
____

Exercise: choose any activity you enjoy that will increase your heart rate to a point where you can answer a question but not carry on a conversation. Average 30 minutes. ____

Breakfast: ____
Snack:____
lunch:____
Snack:____
Dinner: ____

Quiet time: Before bed take 15 minutes to reflect on the day. How did you do? Be kind and forgiving to self and others.

Mind ____
____

Body ____
____

Spirit ____
____

Relationships____
____

Family ____
____

Business____
____

School ____
____

Career ____
____

Day 11

Power thought/quote: ____

What are you thankful for today? ___________________________________

____

____

Quiet time 5-10 minutes: Listen, read, meditate, write daily goals

____

____

____

Exercise: choose any activity you enjoy that will increase your heart rate to a point where you can answer a question but not carry on a conversation. Average 30 minutes. ____

Breakfast: ____

Snack:____

lunch:____

Snack:____

Dinner: ____

Quiet time: Before bed take 15 minutes to reflect on the day. How did you do? Be kind and forgiving to self and others.

Mind ____

____

Body ____

____

Spirit ____

____

Relationships____

____

Family ____

____

Business____

____

School ____

____

Career ____

____

Day 12

Power thought/quote: ____

What are you thankful for today? _______________________________

____

____

Quiet time 5-10 minutes: Listen, read, meditate, write daily goals

____

____

____

Exercise: choose any activity you enjoy that will increase your heart rate to a point where you can answer a question but not carry on a conversation. Average 30 minutes. ____

Breakfast: ____

Snack:____

lunch:____

Snack:____

Dinner: ____

Quiet time: Before bed take 15 minutes to reflect on the day. How did you do? Be kind and forgiving to self and others.

Mind ____

____

Body ____

____

Spirit ____

____

Relationships____

____

Family ____

____

Business____

____

School ____

____

Career ____

____

Day 13

Power thought/quote: _______________________________________

What are you thankful for today? _______________________________
____

Quiet time 5-10 minutes: Listen, read, meditate, write daily goals
____
____
____

Exercise: choose any activity you enjoy that will increase your heart rate to a point where you can answer a question but not carry on a conversation. Average 30 minutes. ____

Breakfast: ____
Snack:____
lunch: ____
Snack:____
Dinner: ____

Quiet time: Before bed take 15 minutes to reflect on the day. How did you do? Be kind and forgiving to self and others.

Mind ____
____

Body ____
____

Spirit ____
____

Relationships____
____

Family ____
____

Business____
____

School ____
____

Career ____
____

Day 14

Power thought/quote: ____

What are you thankful for today? ___________________________________

____

____

Quiet time 5-10 minutes: Listen, read, meditate, write daily goals

____

____

____

Exercise: choose any activity you enjoy that will increase your heart rate to a point where you can answer a question but not carry on a conversation. Average 30 minutes. ____

Breakfast: ____

Snack:____

lunch: ____

Snack:____

Dinner: ____

Quiet time: Before bed take 15 minutes to reflect on the day. How did you do? Be kind and forgiving to self and others.

Mind ____

____

Body ____

____

Spirit ____

____

Relationships____

____

Family ____

____

Business____

____

School ____

____

Career ____

____

Day 15

Power thought/quote:____

What are you thankful for today? ____________________________
____
____

Quiet time 5-10 minutes: Listen, read, meditate, write daily goals
____
____
____

Exercise: choose any activity you enjoy that will increase your heart rate to a point where you can answer a question but not carry on a conversation. Average 30 minutes. ____

Breakfast: ____
Snack:____
lunch:____
Snack:____
Dinner: ____

Quiet time: Before bed take 15 minutes to reflect on the day. How did you do? Be kind and forgiving to self and others.

Mind ____
____

Body ____
____

Spirit ____
____

Relationships____
____

Family ____
____

Business____
____

School ____
____

Career ____
____

Day 16

Power thought/quote: _______________________________________

What are you thankful for today? _______________________________

____

____

Quiet time 5-10 minutes: Listen, read, meditate, write daily goals

____

____

____

Exercise: choose any activity you enjoy that will increase your heart rate to a point where you can answer a question but not carry on a conversation. Average 30 minutes. _______________________________________

Breakfast: ____

Snack:____

lunch:____

Snack:____

Dinner: ____

Quiet time: Before bed take 15 minutes to reflect on the day. How did you do? Be kind and forgiving to self and others.

Mind ____

____

Body ____

____

Spirit ____

____

Relationships____

____

Family ____

____

Business____

____

School ____

____

Career ____

____

Day 17

Power thought/quote: ____

What are you thankful for today? ______________________________________

____

____

Quiet time 5-10 minutes: Listen, read, meditate, write daily goals

____

____

____

Exercise: choose any activity you enjoy that will increase your heart rate to a point where you can answer a question but not carry on a conversation. Average 30 minutes. ____

Breakfast: ____

Snack:____

lunch:____

Snack:____

Dinner: ____

Quiet time: Before bed take 15 minutes to reflect on the day. How did you do? Be kind and forgiving to self and others.

Mind ____

____

Body ____

____

Spirit ____

____

Relationships____

____

Family ____

____

Business____

____

School ____

____

Career ____

____

Day 18

Power thought/quote: _______________________________________

What are you thankful for today? _______________________________
____
____

Quiet time 5-10 minutes: Listen, read, meditate, write daily goals
____
____
____

Exercise: choose any activity you enjoy that will increase your heart rate to a point where you can answer a question but not carry on a conversation. Average 30 minutes. ____

Breakfast: ____
Snack:____
lunch:____
Snack:____
Dinner: ____

Quiet time: Before bed take 15 minutes to reflect on the day. How did you do? Be kind and forgiving to self and others.

Mind ____
____

Body ____
____

Spirit ____
____

Relationships____
____

Family ____
____

Business____
____

School ____
____

Career ____
____

Day 19

Power thought/quote: ____

What are you thankful for today? _______________________________________

____

____

Quiet time 5-10 minutes: Listen, read, meditate, write daily goals

____

____

____

Exercise: choose any activity you enjoy that will increase your heart rate to a point where you can answer a question but not carry on a conversation. Average 30 minutes. ____

Breakfast: ____

Snack:____

lunch:____

Snack:____

Dinner: ____

Quiet time: Before bed take 15 minutes to reflect on the day. How did you do? Be kind and forgiving to self and others.

Mind ____

____

Body ____

____

Spirit ____

____

Relationships____

____

Family ____

____

Business____

____

School ____

____

Career ____

____

Day 20

Power thought/quote: ____

What are you thankful for today? _______________________________________

____

____

Quiet time 5-10 minutes: Listen, read, meditate, write daily goals

____

____

____

Exercise: choose any activity you enjoy that will increase your heart rate to a point where you can answer a question but not carry on a conversation. Average 30 minutes. ____

Breakfast: ____

Snack:____

lunch: ____

Snack:____

Dinner: ____

Quiet time: Before bed take 15 minutes to reflect on the day. How did you do? Be kind and forgiving to self and others.

Mind ____

____

Body ____

____

Spirit ____

____

Relationships____

____

Family ____

____

Business____

____

School ____

____

Career ____

____

Day 21

Power thought/quote: _______________________________________

What are you thankful for today? _______________________________
____
____

Quiet time 5-10 minutes: Listen, read, meditate, write daily goals
____
____
____

Exercise: choose any activity you enjoy that will increase your heart rate to a point where you can answer a question but not carry on a conversation. Average 30 minutes. _______________________________________

Breakfast: ____
Snack:____
lunch: ____
Snack:____
Dinner: ____

Quiet time: Before bed take 15 minutes to reflect on the day. How did you do? Be kind and forgiving to self and others.

Mind ____
____

Body ____
____

Spirit ____
____

Relationships____
____

Family ____
____

Business____
____

School ____
____

Career ____
____

Wow!
Congratulations on your accomplishment. You made it through twenty one days, now this new lifestyle you created should be a habit . Now live the rest of your life with power and purpose

Date / /

Power thought/quote: _______________________________________

What are you thankful for today? _______________________________

____

____

Quiet time 5-10 minutes: Listen, read, meditate, write daily goals

____

____

____

Exercise: choose any activity you enjoy that will increase your heart rate to a point where you can answer a question but not carry on a conversation. Average 30 minutes. _______________________________________

Breakfast: ____

Snack:____

lunch: ____

Snack:____

Dinner: ____

Quiet time: Before bed take 15 minutes to reflect on the day. How did you do? Be kind and forgiving to self and others.

Mind ____

____

Body ____

____

Spirit ____

____

Relationships____

____

Family ____

____

Business____

____

School ____

____

Career ____

____

Date / /

Power thought/quote: _______________________________

What are you thankful for today? _______________________________

____

____

Quiet time 5-10 minutes: Listen, read, meditate, write daily goals

____

____

____

Exercise: choose any activity you enjoy that will increase your heart rate to a point where you can answer a question but not carry on a conversation. Average 30 minutes. _______________________________

Breakfast: _______________________________

Snack:_______________________________

lunch: _______________________________

Snack:_______________________________

Dinner: _______________________________

Quiet time: Before bed take 15 minutes to reflect on the day. How did you do? Be kind and forgiving to self and others.

Mind _______________________________

____

Body _______________________________

____

Spirit _______________________________

____

Relationships_______________________________

____

Family _______________________________

____

Business_______________________________

____

School _______________________________

____

Career _______________________________

____

Date / /

Power thought/quote: ____

What are you thankful for today? ___________________________________

____

____

Quiet time 5-10 minutes: Listen, read, meditate, write daily goals

____

____

____

Exercise: choose any activity you enjoy that will increase your heart rate to a point where you can answer a question but not carry on a conversation. Average 30 minutes. ____

Breakfast: ____

Snack:____

lunch: ____

Snack:____

Dinner: ____

Quiet time: Before bed take 15 minutes to reflect on the day. How did you do? Be kind and forgiving to self and others.

Mind ____

____

Body ____

____

Spirit ____

____

Relationship____

____

Family ____

____

Business____

____

School ____

____

Career ____

____

Date / /

Power thought/quote: _______________________________

What are you thankful for today? _______________________________

____

____

Quiet time 5-10 minutes: Listen, read, meditate, write daily goals

____

____

____

Exercise: choose any activity you enjoy that will increase your heart rate to a point where you can answer a question but not carry on a conversation. Average 30 minutes. _______________________________

Breakfast: _______________________________

Snack:_______________________________

lunch: _______________________________

Snack:_______________________________

Dinner: _______________________________

Quiet time: Before bed take 15 minutes to reflect on the day. How did you do? Be kind and forgiving to self and others.

Mind _______________________________

____

Body _______________________________

____

Spirit _______________________________

____

Relationships_______________________________

____

Family _______________________________

____

Business_______________________________

____

School _______________________________

____

Career _______________________________

____

Date / /

Power thought/quote: ____

What are you thankful for today? _______________________________________
____
____

Quiet time 5-10 minutes: Listen, read, meditate, write daily goals
____
____
____

Exercise: choose any activity you enjoy that will increase your heart rate to a point where you can answer a question but not carry on a conversation. Average 30 minutes. ____

Breakfast: ____
Snack:____
lunch: ____
Snack:____
Dinner: ____

Quiet time: Before bed take 15 minutes to reflect on the day. How did you do? Be kind and forgiving to self and others.

Mind ____
____

Body ____
____

Spirit ____
____

Relationships____
____

Family ____
____

Business____
____

School ____
____

Career ____
____

Date / /

Power thought/quote: _______________________________________

What are you thankful for today? _______________________________
____
____

Quiet time 5-10 minutes: Listen, read, meditate, write daily goals
____
____
____

Exercise: choose any activity you enjoy that will increase your heart rate to a point where you can answer a question but not carry on a conversation. Average 30 minutes. _______________________________________

Breakfast: ____
Snack:____
lunch: ____
Snack:____
Dinner: ____

Quiet time: Before bed take 15 minutes to reflect on the day. How did you do? Be kind and forgiving to self and others.

Mind ____
____

Body ____
____

Spirit ____
____

Relationships____
____

Family ____
____

Business____
____

School ____
____

Career ____
____

Date / /

Power thought/quote: _______________________________________

What are you thankful for today? _______________________________

____

____

Quiet time 5-10 minutes: Listen, read, meditate, write daily goals

____

____

____

Exercise: choose any activity you enjoy that will increase your heart rate to a point where you can answer a question but not carry on a conversation. Average 30 minutes. ____

Breakfast: ____

Snack:____

lunch: ____

Snack:____

Dinner: ____

Quiet time: Before bed take 15 minutes to reflect on the day. How did you do? Be kind and forgiving to self and others.

Mind ____

____

Body ____

____

Spirit ____

____

Relationships____

____

Family ____

____

Business____

____

School ____

____

Career ____

____

Date / /

Power thought/quote: _______________________________________

What are you thankful for today? _______________________________

____

____

Quiet time 5-10 minutes: Listen, read, meditate, write daily goals

____

____

____

Exercise: choose any activity you enjoy that will increase your heart rate to a point where you can answer a question but not carry on a conversation. Average 30 minutes. ____

Breakfast: ____

Snack:____

lunch: ____

Snack:____

Dinner: ____

Quiet time: Before bed take 15 minutes to reflect on the day. How did you do? Be kind and forgiving to self and others.

Mind ____

____

Body ____

____

Spirit ____

____

Relationships____

____

Family ____

____

Business____

____

School ____

____

Career ____

____

Date / /

Power thought/quote: _______________________________________

What are you thankful for today? _______________________________

____

____

Quiet time 5-10 minutes: Listen, read, meditate, write daily goals

____

____

____

Exercise: choose any activity you enjoy that will increase your heart rate to a point where you can answer a question but not carry on a conversation. Average 30 minutes. ____

Breakfast: ____

Snack:____

lunch: ____

Snack:____

Dinner: ____

Quiet time: Before bed take 15 minutes to reflect on the day. How did you do? Be kind and forgiving to self and others.

Mind ____

____

Body ____

____

Spirit ____

____

Relationships____

____

Family ____

____

Business____

____

School ____

____

Career ____

____

Date / /

Power thought/quote: _______________________________

What are you thankful for today? _______________________

____

____

Quiet time 5-10 minutes: Listen, read, meditate, write daily goals

____

____

____

Exercise: choose any activity you enjoy that will increase your heart rate to a point where you can answer a question but not carry on a conversation. Average 30 minutes. ___________________________________

Breakfast: ____

Snack:____

lunch: ____

Snack:____

Dinner: ____

Quiet time: Before bed take 15 minutes to reflect on the day. How did you do? Be kind and forgiving to self and others.

Mind ____

____

Body ____

____

Spirit ____

____

Relationships____

____

Family ____

____

Business____

____

School ____

____

Career ____

____

Date / /

Power thought/quote: ___________________________________

What are you thankful for today? ___________________________

____

____

Quiet time 5-10 minutes: Listen, read, meditate, write daily goals

____

____

____

Exercise: choose any activity you enjoy that will increase your heart rate to a point where you can answer a question but not carry on a conversation. Average 30 minutes. ____

Breakfast: ____

Snack:____

lunch: ____

Snack:____

Dinner: ____

Quiet time: Before bed take 15 minutes to reflect on the day. How did you do? Be kind and forgiving to self and others.

Mind ____

____

Body ____

____

Spirit ____

____

Relationships____

____

Family ____

____

Business____

____

School ____

____

Career ____

____

Date / /

Power thought/quote: _______________________________________

What are you thankful for today? ______________________________

____

____

Quiet time 5-10 minutes: Listen, read, meditate, write daily goals

____

____

____

Exercise: choose any activity you enjoy that will increase your heart rate to a point where you can answer a question but not carry on a conversation. Average 30 minutes. ____

Breakfast: ____

Snack:____

lunch: ____

Snack:____

Dinner: ____

Quiet time: Before bed take 15 minutes to reflect on the day. How did you do? Be kind and forgiving to self and others.

Mind ____

____

Body ____

____

Spirit ____

____

Relationships____

____

Family ____

____

Business____

____

School ____

____

Career ____

____

Date / /

Power thought/quote: _______________________________________

What are you thankful for today? _________________________________
____
____

Quiet time 5-10 minutes: Listen, read, meditate, write daily goals
____
____
____

Exercise: choose any activity you enjoy that will increase your heart rate to a point where you can answer a question but not carry on a conversation. Average 30 minutes. _______________________________________

Breakfast: ____
Snack:____
lunch: ____
Snack:____
Dinner: ____

Quiet time: Before bed take 15 minutes to reflect on the day. How did you do? Be kind and forgiving to self and others.

Mind ____
____

Body ____
____

Spirit ____
____

Relationships____
____

Family ____
____

Business____
____

School ____
____

Career ____
____

Date / /

Power thought/quote: ______________________________

What are you thankful for today? ______________________

____

____

Quiet time 5-10 minutes: Listen, read, meditate, write daily goals

____

____

____

Exercise: choose any activity you enjoy that will increase your heart rate to a point where you can answer a question but not carry on a conversation. Average 30 minutes. ______________________________

Breakfast: ____
Snack:____
lunch: ____
Snack:____
Dinner: ____

Quiet time: Before bed take 15 minutes to reflect on the day. How did you do? Be kind and forgiving to self and others.

Mind ____

____

Body ____

____

Spirit ____

____

Relationships____

____

Family ____

____

Business____

____

School ____

____

Career ____

____

Date / /

Power thought/quote: _______________________________________

What are you thankful for today? ____________________________

____

____

Quiet time 5-10 minutes: Listen, read, meditate, write daily goals

____

____

____

Exercise: choose any activity you enjoy that will increase your heart rate to a point where you can answer a question but not carry on a conversation. Average 30 minutes. ____

Breakfast: ____

Snack:____

lunch: ____

Snack:____

Dinner: ____

Quiet time: Before bed take 15 minutes to reflect on the day. How did you do? Be kind and forgiving to self and others.

Mind ____

____

Body ____

____

Spirit ____

____

Relationships____

____

Family ____

____

Business____

____

School ____

____

Career ____

____

Date / /

Power thought/quote: _______________________________________

What are you thankful for today? _____________________________

____

Quiet time 5-10 minutes: Listen, read, meditate, write daily goals

____

____

____

Exercise: choose any activity you enjoy that will increase your heart rate to a point where you can answer a question but not carry on a conversation. Average 30 minutes. ____________________________________

Breakfast: ____

Snack:____

lunch: ____

Snack:____

Dinner: ____

Quiet time: Before bed take 15 minutes to reflect on the day. How did you do? Be kind and forgiving to self and others.

Mind ____

____

Body ____

____

Spirit ____

____

Relationships____

____

Family ____

____

Business____

____

School ____

____

Career ____

____

Date / /

Power thought/quote: _______________________________________

What are you thankful for today? _______________________________

____

____

Quiet time 5-10 minutes: Listen, read, meditate, write daily goals

____

____

____

Exercise: choose any activity you enjoy that will increase your heart rate to a point where you can answer a question but not carry on a conversation. Average 30 minutes. _______________________________________

Breakfast: ____

Snack:____

lunch: ____

Snack:____

Dinner: ____

Quiet time: Before bed take 15 minutes to reflect on the day. How did you do? Be kind and forgiving to self and others.

Mind ____

____

Body ____

____

Spirit ____

____

Relationships____

____

Family ____

____

Business____

____

School ____

____

Career ____

____

Date / /

Power thought/quote: ___________________________________

What are you thankful for today? _________________________

____

____

Quiet time 5-10 minutes: Listen, read, meditate, write daily goals

____

____

____

Exercise: choose any activity you enjoy that will increase your heart rate to a point where you can answer a question but not carry on a conversation. Average 30 minutes. _________________________________

Breakfast: ____
Snack:____
lunch: ____
Snack:____
Dinner: ____

Quiet time: Before bed take 15 minutes to reflect on the day. How did you do? Be kind and forgiving to self and others.

Mind ____

____

Body ____

____

Spirit ____

____

Relationships____

____

Family ____

____

Business____

____

School ____

____

Career ____

____

Date / /

Power thought/quote: ____

What are you thankful for today? ______________________________________

____

____

Quiet time 5-10 minutes: Listen, read, meditate, write daily goals

____

____

____

Exercise: choose any activity you enjoy that will increase your heart rate to a point where you can answer a question but not carry on a conversation. Average 30 minutes. ____

Breakfast: ____

Snack:____

lunch: ____

Snack:____

Dinner: ____

Quiet time: Before bed take 15 minutes to reflect on the day. How did you do? Be kind and forgiving to self and others.

Mind ____

____

Body ____

____

Spirit ____

____

Relationships____

____

Family ____

____

Business____

____

School ____

____

Career ____

____

Date / /

Power thought/quote: _______________________________

What are you thankful for today? ___________________

____

____

Quiet time 5-10 minutes: Listen, read, meditate, write daily goals

____

____

____

Exercise: choose any activity you enjoy that will increase your heart rate to a point where you can answer a question but not carry on a conversation. Average 30 minutes. _______________________________

Breakfast: ______________________________________

Snack:____

lunch: ____

Snack:____

Dinner: ____

Quiet time: Before bed take 15 minutes to reflect on the day. How did you do? Be kind and forgiving to self and others.

Mind ____

____

Body ____

____

Spirit ____

____

Relationships____________________________________

____

Family ____

____

Business____

____

School ____

____

Career ____

____

Date / /

Power thought/quote: ____

What are you thankful for today? _______________________________________
____
____

Quiet time 5-10 minutes: Listen, read, meditate, write daily goals

____
____
____

Exercise: choose any activity you enjoy that will increase your heart rate to a point where you can answer a question but not carry on a conversation. Average 30 minutes. ____

Breakfast: ____
Snack:____
lunch: ____
Snack:____
Dinner: ____

Quiet time: Before bed take 15 minutes to reflect on the day. How did you do? Be kind and forgiving to self and others.

Mind ____
____

Body ____
____

Spirit ____
____

Relationships____
____

Family ____
____

Business____
____

School ____
____

Career ____
____

Date / /

Power thought/quote: ________________________________

What are you thankful for today? ________________________

____

____

Quiet time 5-10 minutes: Listen, read, meditate, write daily goals

____

____

____

Exercise: choose any activity you enjoy that will increase your heart rate to a point where you can answer a question but not carry on a conversation. Average 30 minutes. ________________________

Breakfast: ____

Snack:____

lunch: ____

Snack:____

Dinner: ____

Quiet time: Before bed take 15 minutes to reflect on the day. How did you do? Be kind and forgiving to self and others.

Mind ____

____

Body ____

____

Spirit ____

____

Relationships_____________________________________

____

Family ____

____

Business____

____

School ____

____

Career ____

____

Date / /

Power thought/quote: ____

What are you thankful for today? ______________________________
____
____

Quiet time 5-10 minutes: Listen, read, meditate, write daily goals
____
____
____

Exercise: choose any activity you enjoy that will increase your heart rate to a point where you can answer a question but not carry on a conversation. Average 30 minutes. ____

Breakfast: ____
Snack:____
lunch: ____
Snack:____
Dinner: ____

Quiet time: Before bed take 15 minutes to reflect on the day. How did you do? Be kind and forgiving to self and others.

Mind ____
____

Body ____
____

Spirit ____
____

Relationships____
____

Family ____
____

Business____
____

School ____
____

Career ____
____

Date / /

Power thought/quote: _______________________________________

What are you thankful for today? _______________________________

____

____

Quiet time 5-10 minutes: Listen, read, meditate, write daily goals

____

____

____

Exercise: choose any activity you enjoy that will increase your heart rate to a point where you can answer a question but not carry on a conversation. Average 30 minutes. ____

Breakfast: ____

Snack:____

lunch: ____

Snack:____

Dinner: ____

Quiet time: Before bed take 15 minutes to reflect on the day. How did you do? Be kind and forgiving to self and others.

Mind ____

____

Body ____

____

Spirit ____

____

Relationships____

____

Family ____

____

Business____

____

School ____

____

Career ____

____

Date / /

Power thought/quote: ____

What are you thankful for today? _______________________________

____

____

Quiet time 5-10 minutes: Listen, read, meditate, write daily goals

____

____

____

Exercise: choose any activity you enjoy that will increase your heart rate to a point where you can answer a question but not carry on a conversation. Average 30 minutes. ____

Breakfast: ____

Snack:____

lunch: ____

Snack:____

Dinner: ____

Quiet time: Before bed take 15 minutes to reflect on the day. How did you do? Be kind and forgiving to self and others.

Mind ____

____

Body ____

____

Spirit ____

____

Relationships____

____

Family ____

____

Business____

____

School ____

____

Career ____

____

Date / /

Power thought/quote: _______________________________________

What are you thankful for today? _______________________________

____

____

Quiet time 5-10 minutes: Listen, read, meditate, write daily goals

____

____

____

Exercise: choose any activity you enjoy that will increase your heart rate to a point where you can answer a question but not carry on a conversation. Average 30 minutes. ____

Breakfast: ____
Snack:____
lunch: ____
Snack:____
Dinner: ____

Quiet time: Before bed take 15 minutes to reflect on the day. How did you do? Be kind and forgiving to self and others.

Mind ____

____

Body ____

____

Spirit ____

____

Relationships____

____

Family ____

____

Business____

____

School ____

____

Career ____

____

Date / /

Power thought/quote: _______________________________________

What are you thankful for today? ____________________________

____

____

Quiet time 5-10 minutes: Listen, read, meditate, write daily goals

____

____

____

Exercise: choose any activity you enjoy that will increase your heart rate to a point where you can answer a question but not carry on a conversation. Average 30 minutes. ____

Breakfast: ____

Snack:____

lunch: ____

Snack:____

Dinner: ____

Quiet time: Before bed take 15 minutes to reflect on the day. How did you do? Be kind and forgiving to self and others.

Mind ____

____

Body ____

____

Spirit ____

____

Relationships____

____

Family ____

____

Business____

____

School ____

____

Career ____

____

Date / /

Power thought/quote: _______________________________________

What are you thankful for today? _______________________________

____

____

Quiet time 5-10 minutes: Listen, read, meditate, write daily goals

____

____

____

Exercise: choose any activity you enjoy that will increase your heart rate to a point where you can answer a question but not carry on a conversation. Average 30 minutes. _______________________________________

Breakfast: ____

Snack:____

lunch: ____

Snack:____

Dinner: ____

Quiet time: Before bed take 15 minutes to reflect on the day. How did you do? Be kind and forgiving to self and others.

Mind ____

____

Body ____

____

Spirit ____

____

Relationships____

____

Family ____

____

Business____

____

School ____

____

Career ____

____

Date / /

Power thought/quote: _______________________________________

What are you thankful for today? _______________________________
____
____

Quiet time 5-10 minutes: Listen, read, meditate, write daily goals
____
____
____

Exercise: choose any activity you enjoy that will increase your heart rate to a point where you can answer a question but not carry on a conversation. Average 30 minutes. ____

Breakfast: ____
Snack:____
lunch: ____
Snack:____
Dinner: ____

Quiet time: Before bed take 15 minutes to reflect on the day. How did you do? Be kind and forgiving to self and others.

Mind ____
____

Body ____
____

Spirit ____
____

Relationships____
____

Family ____
____

Business____
____

School ____
____

Career ____
____

Date / /

Power thought/quote: ____

What are you thankful for today? _________________________________

____

____

Quiet time 5-10 minutes: Listen, read, meditate, write daily goals

____

____

____

Exercise: choose any activity you enjoy that will increase your heart rate to a point where you can answer a question but not carry on a conversation. Average 30 minutes. ____

Breakfast: ____

Snack:____

lunch: ____

Snack:____

Dinner: ____

Quiet time: Before bed take 15 minutes to reflect on the day. How did you do? Be kind and forgiving to self and others.

Mind ____

____

Body ____

____

Spirit ____

____

Realtionships____

____

Family ____

____

Business____

____

School ____

____

Career ____

____

Date / /

Power thought/quote: ____

What are you thankful for today? ________________________________

____

____

Quiet time 5-10 minutes: Listen, read, meditate, write daily goals

____

____

____

Exercise: choose any activity you enjoy that will increase your heart rate to a point where you can answer a question but not carry on a conversation. Average 30 minutes. ____

Breakfast: ____

Snack:____

lunch: ____

Snack:____

Dinner: ____

Quiet time: Before bed take 15 minutes to reflect on the day. How did you do? Be kind and forgiving to self and others.

Mind ____

____

Body ____

____

Spirit ____

____

Relationships____

____

Family ____

____

Business____

____

School ____

____

Career ____

____

Date / /

Power thought/quote: _______________________________

What are you thankful for today? _______________________________

____

____

Quiet time 5-10 minutes: Listen, read, meditate, write daily goals

____

____

____

Exercise: choose any activity you enjoy that will increase your heart rate to a point where you can answer a question but not carry on a conversation. Average 30 minutes. _______________________________

Breakfast: _______________________________

Snack:_______________________________

lunch: _______________________________

Snack:_______________________________

Dinner: _______________________________

Quiet time: Before bed take 15 minutes to reflect on the day. How did you do? Be kind and forgiving to self and others.

Mind _______________________________

____

Body _______________________________

____

Spirit _______________________________

____

Relationships_______________________________

____

Family _______________________________

____

Business_______________________________

____

School _______________________________

____

Career _______________________________

____

Date / /

Power thought/quote: _______________________________________

What are you thankful for today? _______________________________

____

____

Quiet time 5-10 minutes: Listen, read, meditate, write daily goals

____

____

____

Exercise: choose any activity you enjoy that will increase your heart rate to a point where you can answer a question but not carry on a conversation. Average 30 minutes. _______________________________________

Breakfast: ____

Snack:____

lunch: ____

Snack:____

Dinner: ____

Quiet time: Before bed take 15 minutes to reflect on the day. How did you do? Be kind and forgiving to self and others.

Mind ____

____

Body ____

____

Spirit ____

____

Relationships____

____

Family ____

____

Business____

____

School ____

____

Career ____

____

Date / /

Power thought/quote: _________________________________

What are you thankful for today? _________________________

____

____

Quiet time 5-10 minutes: Listen, read, meditate, write daily goals

____

____

____

Exercise: choose any activity you enjoy that will increase your heart rate to a point where you can answer a question but not carry on a conversation. Average 30 minutes. ____

Breakfast: _______________________________________

Snack:____

lunch: ____

Snack:____

Dinner: ____

Quiet time: Before bed take 15 minutes to reflect on the day. How did you do? Be kind and forgiving to self and others.

Mind ____

____

Body ____

____

Spirit ____

____

Relationships______________________________________

____

Family ____

____

Business____

____

School ____

____

Career ____

____

Date / /

Power thought/quote: _______________________________________

What are you thankful for today? _______________________________

____

____

Quiet time 5-10 minutes: Listen, read, meditate, write daily goals

____

____

____

Exercise: choose any activity you enjoy that will increase your heart rate to a point where you can answer a question but not carry on a conversation. Average 30 minutes. ____

Breakfast: ____

Snack:____

lunch: ____

Snack:____

Dinner: ____

Quiet time: Before bed take 15 minutes to reflect on the day. How did you do? Be kind and forgiving to self and others.

Mind ____

____

Body ____

____

Spirit ____

____

Relationships____

____

Family ____

____

Business____

____

School ____

____

Career ____

____

Date / /

Power thought/quote: ______________________________________

What are you thankful for today? ______________________________
____
____

Quiet time 5-10 minutes: Listen, read, meditate, write daily goals

____
____
____

Exercise: choose any activity you enjoy that will increase your heart rate to a point where you can answer a question but not carry on a conversation. Average 30 minutes. ____

Breakfast: ____
Snack:____
lunch: ____
Snack:____
Dinner: ____

Quiet time: Before bed take 15 minutes to reflect on the day. How did you do? Be kind and forgiving to self and others.

Mind ____
____

Body ____
____

Spirit ____
____

Relationships____
____

Family ____
____

Business____
____

School ____
____

Career ____
____

Date / /

Power thought/quote: _______________________________________

What are you thankful for today? _______________________________

____

____

Quiet time 5-10 minutes: Listen, read, meditate, write daily goals

____

____

____

Exercise: choose any activity you enjoy that will increase your heart rate to a point where you can answer a question but not carry on a conversation. Average 30 minutes. _______________________________________

Breakfast: ____

Snack:____

lunch: ____

Snack:____

Dinner: ____

Quiet time: Before bed take 15 minutes to reflect on the day. How did you do? Be kind and forgiving to self and others.

Mind ____

____

Body ____

____

Spirit ____

____

Relationships____

____

Family ____

____

Business____

____

School ____

____

Career ____

____

Date / /

Power thought/quote: _______________________________

What are you thankful for today? _______________________

____

____

Quiet time 5-10 minutes: Listen, read, meditate, write daily goals

____

____

____

Exercise: choose any activity you enjoy that will increase your heart rate to a point where you can answer a question but not carry on a conversation. Average 30 minutes. _______________________________

Breakfast: _____________________________________

Snack:____

lunch: ____

Snack:____

Dinner: _______________________________________

Quiet time: Before bed take 15 minutes to reflect on the day. How did you do? Be kind and forgiving to self and others.

Mind ____

____

Body ____

____

Spirit ____

____

Relationships___________________________________

____

Family ____

____

Business_______________________________________

____

School ____

____

Career ____

____

Date / /

Power thought/quote: _______________________________________

What are you thankful for today? _______________________________

____

____

Quiet time 5-10 minutes: Listen, read, meditate, write daily goals

____

____

____

Exercise: choose any activity you enjoy that will increase your heart rate to a point where you can answer a question but not carry on a conversation. Average 30 minutes. ____

Breakfast: ____

Snack:____

lunch: ____

Snack:____

Dinner: ____

Quiet time: Before bed take 15 minutes to reflect on the day. How did you do? Be kind and forgiving to self and others.

Mind ____

____

Body ____

____

Spirit ____

____

Relationships____

____

Family ____

____

Business____

____

School ____

____

Career ____

____

Date / /

Power thought/quote: _______________________________

What are you thankful for today? _______________________

____

____

Quiet time 5-10 minutes: Listen, read, meditate, write daily goals

____

____

____

Exercise: choose any activity you enjoy that will increase your heart rate to a point where you can answer a question but not carry on a conversation. Average 30 minutes. _______________________________

Breakfast: _____________________________________

Snack:____

lunch: ____

Snack:____

Dinner: _______________________________________

Quiet time: Before bed take 15 minutes to reflect on the day. How did you do? Be kind and forgiving to self and others.

Mind ____

____

Body ____

____

Spirit ____

____

Relationships___________________________________

____

Family ____

____

Business_______________________________________

____

School ____

____

Career ____

____

Date / /

Power thought/quote: ____

What are you thankful for today? _______________________________________

____

____

Quiet time 5-10 minutes: Listen, read, meditate, write daily goals

____

____

____

Exercise: choose any activity you enjoy that will increase your heart rate to a point where you can answer a question but not carry on a conversation. Average 30 minutes. ____

Breakfast: ____

Snack:____

lunch: ____

Snack:____

Dinner: ____

Quiet time: Before bed take 15 minutes to reflect on the day. How did you do? Be kind and forgiving to self and others.

Mind ____

____

Body ____

____

Spirit ____

____

Relationships____

____

Family ____

____

Business____

____

School ____

____

Career ____

____

Date / /

Power thought/quote: _______________________________________

What are you thankful for today? _____________________________

____

____

Quiet time 5-10 minutes: Listen, read, meditate, write daily goals

____

____

____

Exercise: choose any activity you enjoy that will increase your heart rate to a point where you can answer a question but not carry on a conversation. Average 30 minutes. ____

Breakfast: ____

Snack:____

lunch: ____

Snack:____

Dinner: ____

Quiet time: Before bed take 15 minutes to reflect on the day. How did you do? Be kind and forgiving to self and others.

Mind____

____

Body____

____

Spirit____

____

Relationships____

____

Family____

____

Business____

____

School____

____

Career____

____

Date / /

Power thought/quote: _______________________________________

What are you thankful for today? ___________________________
____
____

Quiet time 5-10 minutes: Listen, read, meditate, write daily goals
____
____
____

Exercise: choose any activity you enjoy that will increase your heart rate to a point where you can answer a question but not carry on a conversation. Average 30 minutes. ____

Breakfast: ____
Snack:____
lunch: ____
Snack:____
Dinner: ____

Quiet time: Before bed take 15 minutes to reflect on the day. How did you do? Be kind and forgiving to self and others.

Mind ____
____

Body ____
____

Spirit ____
____

Relationships____
____

Family ____
____

Business____
____

School ____
____

Career ____
____

Date / /

Power thought/quote: _______________________________________

What are you thankful for today? _______________________________

____

____

Quiet time 5-10 minutes: Listen, read, meditate, write daily goals

____

____

____

Exercise: choose any activity you enjoy that will increase your heart rate to a point where you can answer a question but not carry on a conversation. Average 30 minutes. ____

Breakfast: ____

Snack:____

lunch: ____

Snack:____

Dinner: ____

Quiet time: Before bed take 15 minutes to reflect on the day. How did you do? Be kind and forgiving to self and others.

Mind ____

____

Body ____

____

Spirit ____

____

Relationships____

____

Family ____

____

Business____

____

School ____

____

Career ____

____

Date / /

Power thought/quote: _______________________________________

What are you thankful for today? _______________________________
____
____

Quiet time 5-10 minutes: Listen, read, meditate, write daily goals
____
____
____

Exercise: choose any activity you enjoy that will increase your heart rate to a point where you can answer a question but not carry on a conversation. Average 30 minutes. ____

Breakfast: ____
Snack:____
lunch: ____
Snack:____
Dinner: ____

Quiet time: Before bed take 15 minutes to reflect on the day. How did you do? Be kind and forgiving to self and others.

Mind ____
____

Body ____
____

Spirit ____
____

Relationships____
____

Family ____
____

Business____
____

School ____
____

Career ____
____

Date / /

Power thought/quote: _______________________________________

What are you thankful for today? _______________________________

____

____

Quiet time 5-10 minutes: Listen, read, meditate, write daily goals

____

____

____

Exercise: choose any activity you enjoy that will increase your heart rate to a point where you can answer a question but not carry on a conversation. Average 30 minutes. ____

Breakfast: ____

Snack:____

lunch: ____

Snack:____

Dinner: ____

Quiet time: Before bed take 15 minutes to reflect on the day. How did you do? Be kind and forgiving to self and others.

Mind ____

____

Body ____

____

Spirit ____

____

Relationships____

____

Family ____

____

Business____

____

School ____

____

Career ____

____

Date / /

Power thought/quote: ____

What are you thankful for today? ________________________________
____
____

Quiet time 5-10 minutes: Listen, read, meditate, write daily goals
____
____
____

Exercise: choose any activity you enjoy that will increase your heart rate to a point where you can answer a question but not carry on a conversation. Average 30 minutes. ____

Breakfast: ____
Snack:____
lunch: ____
Snack:____
Dinner: ____

Quiet time: Before bed take 15 minutes to reflect on the day. How did you do? Be kind and forgiving to self and others.

Mind ____
____

Body ____
____

Spirit ____
____

Relationships____
____

Family ____
____

Business____
____

School ____
____

Career ____
____

Date / /

Power thought/quote: _______________________________________

What are you thankful for today? ___________________________

____

____

Quiet time 5-10 minutes: Listen, read, meditate, write daily goals

____

____

____

Exercise: choose any activity you enjoy that will increase your heart rate to a point where you can answer a question but not carry on a conversation. Average 30 minutes. ____

Breakfast: ____
Snack:____
lunch: ____
Snack:____
Dinner: ____

Quiet time: Before bed take 15 minutes to reflect on the day. How did you do? Be kind and forgiving to self and others.

Mind ____

____

Body ____

____

Spirit ____

____

Relationships____

____

Family ____

____

Business____

____

School ____

____

Career ____

____

Date / /

Power thought/quote: _______________________________________

What are you thankful for today? _______________________________

____

____

Quiet time 5-10 minutes: Listen, read, meditate, write daily goals

____

____

____

Exercise: choose any activity you enjoy that will increase your heart rate to a point where you can answer a question but not carry on a conversation. Average 30 minutes. _______________________________________

Breakfast: _______________________________________

Snack:_______________________________________

lunch: _______________________________________

Snack:_______________________________________

Dinner: _______________________________________

Quiet time: Before bed take 15 minutes to reflect on the day. How did you do? Be kind and forgiving to self and others.

Mind _______________________________________

____

Body _______________________________________

____

Spirit _______________________________________

____

Relationships_______________________________________

____

Family _______________________________________

____

Business_______________________________________

____

School _______________________________________

____

Career _______________________________________

____

Date / /

Power thought/quote: _______________________________

What are you thankful for today? _______________________

____

____

Quiet time 5-10 minutes: Listen, read, meditate, write daily goals

____

____

____

Exercise: choose any activity you enjoy that will increase your heart rate to a point where you can answer a question but not carry on a conversation. Average 30 minutes. _________________________

Breakfast: _____________________________________

Snack:____

lunch: ____

Snack:____

Dinner: ____

Quiet time: Before bed take 15 minutes to reflect on the day. How did you do? Be kind and forgiving to self and others.

Mind ____

____

Body ____

____

Spirit ____

____

Relationships____________________________________

____

Family ____

____

Business_______________________________________

____

School ____

____

Career ____

____

Date / /

Power thought/quote: _______________________________________

What are you thankful for today? _______________________________
____
____

Quiet time 5-10 minutes: Listen, read, meditate, write daily goals

____
____
____

Exercise: choose any activity you enjoy that will increase your heart rate to a point where you can answer a question but not carry on a conversation. Average 30 minutes. _______________________________________

Breakfast: _______________________________________
Snack:_______________________________________
lunch: _______________________________________
Snack:_______________________________________
Dinner: _______________________________________

Quiet time: Before bed take 15 minutes to reflect on the day. How did you do? Be kind and forgiving to self and others.

Mind _______________________________________
____

Body _______________________________________
____

Spirit _______________________________________
____

Relationships_______________________________________
____

Family _______________________________________
____

Business_______________________________________
____

School _______________________________________
____

Career _______________________________________
____

Date / /

Power thought/quote: _______________________________

What are you thankful for today? _______________________________

____

____

Quiet time 5-10 minutes: Listen, read, meditate, write daily goals

____

____

____

Exercise: choose any activity you enjoy that will increase your heart rate to a point where you can answer a question but not carry on a conversation. Average 30 minutes. _______________________________

Breakfast: _______________________________

Snack:_______________________________

lunch: _______________________________

Snack:_______________________________

Dinner: _______________________________

Quiet time: Before bed take 15 minutes to reflect on the day. How did you do? Be kind and forgiving to self and others.

Mind _______________________________

____

Body _______________________________

____

Spirit _______________________________

____

Relationships_______________________________

____

Family _______________________________

____

Business_______________________________

____

School _______________________________

____

Career _______________________________

____

Date / /

Power thought/quote: ____

What are you thankful for today? ______________________________________
____
____

Quiet time 5-10 minutes: Listen, read, meditate, write daily goals

____
____
____

Exercise: choose any activity you enjoy that will increase your heart rate to a point where you can answer a question but not carry on a conversation. Average 30 minutes. ____

Breakfast: ____
Snack:____
lunch: ____
Snack:____
Dinner: ____

Quiet time: Before bed take 15 minutes to reflect on the day. How did you do? Be kind and forgiving to self and others.

Mind ____
____

Body ____
____

Spirit ____
____

Relationships____
____

Family ____
____

Business____
____

School ____
____

Career ____
____

Date / /

Power thought/quote: _______________________________

What are you thankful for today? _______________________
____
____

Quiet time 5-10 minutes: Listen, read, meditate, write daily goals
____
____
____

Exercise: choose any activity you enjoy that will increase your heart rate to a point where you can answer a question but not carry on a conversation. Average 30 minutes. ____________________________________

Breakfast: ______________________________________
Snack:____
lunch: ____
Snack:____
Dinner: ____

Quiet time: Before bed take 15 minutes to reflect on the day. How did you do? Be kind and forgiving to self and others.

Mind ____
____

Body____
____

Spirit ____
____

Relationships_____________________________________
____

Family ____
____

Business____
____

School ____
____

Career ____
____

Date / /

Power thought/quote: ___________________________________

What are you thankful for today? ___________________________
____
____

Quiet time 5-10 minutes: Listen, read, meditate, write daily goals
____
____
____

Exercise: choose any activity you enjoy that will increase your heart rate to a point where you can answer a question but not carry on a conversation. Average 30 minutes. _______________________________________

Breakfast: ____
Snack:____
lunch: ____
Snack:____
Dinner: ____

Quiet time: Before bed take 15 minutes to reflect on the day. How did you do? Be kind and forgiving to self and others.

Mind ____
____

Body ____
____

Spirit ____
____

Relationships_______________________________________
____

Family ____
____

Business____
____

School ____
____

Career ____
____

Date / /

Power thought/quote: ________________________________

What are you thankful for today? ________________________

____

____

Quiet time 5-10 minutes: Listen, read, meditate, write daily goals

____

____

____

Exercise: choose any activity you enjoy that will increase your heart rate to a point where you can answer a question but not carry on a conversation. Average 30 minutes. ________________________

Breakfast: ________________________________

Snack:____________________________________

lunch: ___________________________________

Snack:____________________________________

Dinner: __________________________________

Quiet time: Before bed take 15 minutes to reflect on the day. How did you do? Be kind and forgiving to self and others.

Mind ________________________________

____

Body ________________________________

____

Spirit ________________________________

____

Relationships________________________________

____

Family ________________________________

____

Business________________________________

____

School ________________________________

____

Career ________________________________

____

Date / /

Power thought/quote: _______________________________________

What are you thankful for today? _______________________________________

____

____

Quiet time 5-10 minutes: Listen, read, meditate, write daily goals

____

____

____

Exercise: choose any activity you enjoy that will increase your heart rate to a point where you can answer a question but not carry on a conversation. Average 30 minutes. _______________________________________

Breakfast: _______________________________________

Snack:_______________________________________

lunch: _______________________________________

Snack:_______________________________________

Dinner: _______________________________________

Quiet time: Before bed take 15 minutes to reflect on the day. How did you do? Be kind and forgiving to self and others.

Mind _______________________________________

____

Body _______________________________________

____

Spirit _______________________________________

____

Relationships_______________________________________

____

Family _______________________________________

____

Business_______________________________________

____

School _______________________________________

____

Career _______________________________________

____

Date / /

Power thought/quote: _______________________________________

What are you thankful for today? _______________________________
____
____

Quiet time 5-10 minutes: Listen, read, meditate, write daily goals

____
____
____

Exercise: choose any activity you enjoy that will increase your heart rate to a point where you can answer a question but not carry on a conversation. Average 30 minutes. _______________________________________

Breakfast: ____
Snack:____
lunch: ____
Snack:____
Dinner: ____

Quiet time: Before bed take 15 minutes to reflect on the day. How did you do? Be kind and forgiving to self and others.

Mind ____
____

Body ____
____

Spirit ____
____

Relationships____
____

Family ____
____

Business____
____

School ____
____

Career ____
____

Date / /

Power thought/quote: ____

What are you thankful for today? _______________________________________
____
____

Quiet time 5-10 minutes: Listen, read, meditate, write daily goals
____
____
____

Exercise: choose any activity you enjoy that will increase your heart rate to a point where you can answer a question but not carry on a conversation. Average 30 minutes. ____

Breakfast: ____
Snack:____
lunch: ____
Snack:____
Dinner: ____

Quiet time: Before bed take 15 minutes to reflect on the day. How did you do? Be kind and forgiving to self and others.

Mind ____
____

Body ____
____

Spirit ____
____

Relationships____
____

Family ____
____

Business____
____

School ____
____

Career ____
____

Date / /

Power thought/quote: _______________________________________

What are you thankful for today? _______________________________
____
____

Quiet time 5-10 minutes: Listen, read, meditate, write daily goals
____
____
____

Exercise: choose any activity you enjoy that will increase your heart rate to a point where you can answer a question but not carry on a conversation. Average 30 minutes. _______________________________________

Breakfast: ____
Snack:____
lunch: ____
Snack:____
Dinner: ____

Quiet time: Before bed take 15 minutes to reflect on the day. How did you do? Be kind and forgiving to self and others.

Mind ____
____

Body ____
____

Spirit ____
____

Relationships____
____

Family ____
____

Business____
____

School ____
____

Career ____
____

Date / /

Power thought/quote: _______________________________

What are you thankful for today? _______________________________
____
____

Quiet time 5-10 minutes: Listen, read, meditate, write daily goals
____
____
____

Exercise: choose any activity you enjoy that will increase your heart rate to a point where you can answer a question but not carry on a conversation. Average 30 minutes. _______________________________

Breakfast: _______________________________
Snack:_______________________________
lunch: _______________________________
Snack:_______________________________
Dinner: _______________________________

Quiet time: Before bed take 15 minutes to reflect on the day. How did you do? Be kind and forgiving to self and others.

Mind _______________________________
____

Body _______________________________
____

Spirit _______________________________
____

Relationships_______________________________
____

Family _______________________________
____

Business_______________________________
____

School _______________________________
____

Career _______________________________
____

Date / /

Power thought/quote: _______________________________________

What are you thankful for today? _______________________________

____

Quiet time 5-10 minutes: Listen, read, meditate, write daily goals

____

____

____

Exercise: choose any activity you enjoy that will increase your heart rate to a point where you can answer a question but not carry on a conversation. Average 30 minutes. ____

Breakfast: ____

Snack:____

lunch: ____

Snack:____

Dinner: ____

Quiet time: Before bed take 15 minutes to reflect on the day. How did you do? Be kind and forgiving to self and others.

Mind ____

____

Body ____

____

Spirit ____

____

Relationships____

____

Family ____

____

Business____

____

School ____

____

Career ____

____

Date / /

Power thought/quote: _______________________________________

What are you thankful for today? _______________________________

____

____

Quiet time 5-10 minutes: Listen, read, meditate, write daily goals

____

____

____

Exercise: choose any activity you enjoy that will increase your heart rate to a point where you can answer a question but not carry on a conversation. Average 30 minutes. _______________________________________

Breakfast: ____

Snack:____

lunch: ____

Snack:____

Dinner: ____

Quiet time: Before bed take 15 minutes to reflect on the day. How did you do? Be kind and forgiving to self and others.

Mind ____

____

Body ____

____

Spirit ____

____

Relationships____

____

Family ____

____

Business____

____

School ____

____

Career ____

____

Date / /

Power thought/quote: _______________________________

What are you thankful for today? _______________________________

____

____

Quiet time 5-10 minutes: Listen, read, meditate, write daily goals

____

____

____

Exercise: choose any activity you enjoy that will increase your heart rate to a point where you can answer a question but not carry on a conversation. Average 30 minutes. _______________________________

Breakfast: _______________________________

Snack:_______________________________

lunch: _______________________________

Snack:_______________________________

Dinner: _______________________________

Quiet time: Before bed take 15 minutes to reflect on the day. How did you do? Be kind and forgiving to self and others.

Mind _______________________________

____

Body _______________________________

____

Spirit _______________________________

____

Relationships_______________________________

____

Family _______________________________

____

Business_______________________________

____

School _______________________________

____

Career _______________________________

____

Date / /

Power thought/quote: _______________________________________

What are you thankful for today? _______________________________

____

____

Quiet time 5-10 minutes: Listen, read, meditate, write daily goals

____

____

____

Exercise: choose any activity you enjoy that will increase your heart rate to a point where you can answer a question but not carry on a conversation. Average 30 minutes. ____

Breakfast: ____

Snack:____

lunch: ____

Snack:____

Dinner: ____

Quiet time: Before bed take 15 minutes to reflect on the day. How did you do? Be kind and forgiving to self and others.

Mind ____

____

Body ____

____

Spirit ____

____

Relationships____

____

Family ____

____

Business____

____

School ____

____

Career ____

____

Date / /

Power thought/quote: _______________________________________

What are you thankful for today? _______________________________

____

____

Quiet time 5-10 minutes: Listen, read, meditate, write daily goals

____

____

____

Exercise: choose any activity you enjoy that will increase your heart rate to a point where you can answer a question but not carry on a conversation. Average 30 minutes. ____

Breakfast: ____

Snack:____

lunch: ____

Snack:____

Dinner: ____

Quiet time: Before bed take 15 minutes to reflect on the day. How did you do? Be kind and forgiving to self and others.

Mind ____

____

Body ____

____

Spirit ____

____

Relationships____

____

Family ____

____

Business____

____

School ____

____

Career ____

____

Date / /

Power thought/quote: ____

What are you thankful for today? _______________________________________
____

Quiet time 5-10 minutes: Listen, read, meditate, write daily goals

____
____
____

Exercise: choose any activity you enjoy that will increase your heart rate to a point where you can answer a question but not carry on a conversation. Average 30 minutes. ____

Breakfast: ____
Snack:____
lunch: ____
Snack:____
Dinner: ____

Quiet time: Before bed take 15 minutes to reflect on the day. How did you do? Be kind and forgiving to self and others.

Mind ____
____

Body ____
____

Spirit ____
____

Relationships____
____

Family ____
____

Business____
____

School ____
____

Career ____
____

Date / /

Power thought/quote: _______________________________________

What are you thankful for today? _____________________________
____
____

Quiet time 5-10 minutes: Listen, read, meditate, write daily goals
____
____
____

Exercise: choose any activity you enjoy that will increase your heart rate to a point where you can answer a question but not carry on a conversation. Average 30 minutes. ____

Breakfast: ____
Snack:____
lunch: ____
Snack:____
Dinner: ____

Quiet time: Before bed take 15 minutes to reflect on the day. How did you do? Be kind and forgiving to self and others.

Mind ____
____

Body ____
____

Spirit ____
____

Relationships____
____

Family ____
____

Business____
____

School ____
____

Career ____
____

Date / /

Power thought/quote: ____

What are you thankful for today? _______________________________________

____

____

Quiet time 5-10 minutes: Listen, read, meditate, write daily goals

____

____

____

Exercise: choose any activity you enjoy that will increase your heart rate to a point where you can answer a question but not carry on a conversation. Average 30 minutes. ____

Breakfast: ____

Snack:____

lunch: ____

Snack:____

Dinner: ____

Quiet time: Before bed take 15 minutes to reflect on the day. How did you do? Be kind and forgiving to self and others.

Mind ____

____

Body ____

____

Spirit ____

____

Relationships____

____

Family ____

____

Business____

____

School ____

____

Career ____

____

Date / /

Power thought/quote: _______________________________________

What are you thankful for today? _______________________________

____

____

Quiet time 5-10 minutes: Listen, read, meditate, write daily goals

____

____

____

Exercise: choose any activity you enjoy that will increase your heart rate to a point where you can answer a question but not carry on a conversation. Average 30 minutes. ____

Breakfast: ____

Snack:____

lunch: ____

Snack:____

Dinner: ____

Quiet time: Before bed take 15 minutes to reflect on the day. How did you do? Be kind and forgiving to self and others.

Mind ____

____

Body ____

____

Spirit ____

____

Relationships____

____

Family ____

____

Business____

____

School ____

____

Career ____

____

Date / /

Power thought/quote: _______________________________________

What are you thankful for today? _______________________________

____

____

Quiet time 5-10 minutes: Listen, read, meditate, write daily goals

____

____

____

Exercise: choose any activity you enjoy that will increase your heart rate to a point where you can answer a question but not carry on a conversation. Average 30 minutes. _______________________________________

Breakfast: ____

Snack:____

lunch: ____

Snack:____

Dinner: ____

Quiet time: Before bed take 15 minutes to reflect on the day. How did you do? Be kind and forgiving to self and others.

Mind ____

____

Body ____

____

Spirit ____

____

Relationships____

____

Family ____

____

Business____

____

School ____

____

Career ____

____

Date / /

Power thought/quote: ________________________________

What are you thankful for today? ________________________

____

____

Quiet time 5-10 minutes: Listen, read, meditate, write daily goals

____

____

____

Exercise: choose any activity you enjoy that will increase your heart rate to a point where you can answer a question but not carry on a conversation. Average 30 minutes. ______________________________________

Breakfast: ____
Snack:____
lunch: ____
Snack:____
Dinner: ____

Quiet time: Before bed take 15 minutes to reflect on the day. How did you do? Be kind and forgiving to self and others.

Mind ____

____

Body ____

____

Spirit ____

____

Relationships____

____

Family ____

____

Business____

____

School ____

____

Career ____

____

Date / /

Power thought/quote: ____

What are you thankful for today? ______________________________________

____

____

Quiet time 5-10 minutes: Listen, read, meditate, write daily goals

____

____

____

Exercise: choose any activity you enjoy that will increase your heart rate to a point where you can answer a question but not carry on a conversation. Average 30 minutes. ____

Breakfast: ____

Snack:____

lunch: ____

Snack:____

Dinner: ____

Quiet time: Before bed take 15 minutes to reflect on the day. How did you do? Be kind and forgiving to self and others.

Mind ____

____

Body ____

____

Spirit ____

____

Relationships____

____

Family ____

____

Business____

____

School ____

____

Career ____

____

Date / /

Power thought/quote: _______________________________

What are you thankful for today? _______________________
____
____

Quiet time 5-10 minutes: Listen, read, meditate, write daily goals
____
____
____

Exercise: choose any activity you enjoy that will increase your heart rate to a point where you can answer a question but not carry on a conversation. Average 30 minutes. ___________________________________

Breakfast: ____
Snack:____
lunch: ____
Snack:____
Dinner: ____

Quiet time: Before bed take 15 minutes to reflect on the day. How did you do? Be kind and forgiving to self and others.

Mind ____
____

Body ____
____

Spirit ____
____

Relationships____
____

Family ____
____

Business____
____

School ____
____

Career ____
____

Date / /

Power thought/quote: _______________________________________

What are you thankful for today? _______________________________
____
____

Quiet time 5-10 minutes: Listen, read, meditate, write daily goals

____
____
____

Exercise: choose any activity you enjoy that will increase your heart rate to a point where you can answer a question but not carry on a conversation. Average 30 minutes. ____

Breakfast: ____
Snack:____
lunch: ____
Snack:____
Dinner: ____

Quiet time: Before bed take 15 minutes to reflect on the day. How did you do? Be kind and forgiving to self and others.

Mind ____
____

Body ____
____

Spirit ____
____

Relationships____
____

Family ____
____

Business____
____

School ____
____

Career ____
____

Date / /

Power thought/quote: ___________________________________

What are you thankful for today? _________________________

____

____

Quiet time 5-10 minutes: Listen, read, meditate, write daily goals

____

____

____

Exercise: choose any activity you enjoy that will increase your heart rate to a point where you can answer a question but not carry on a conversation. Average 30 minutes. ______________________________________

Breakfast: ____

Snack:____

lunch: ____

Snack:____

Dinner: ____

Quiet time: Before bed take 15 minutes to reflect on the day. How did you do? Be kind and forgiving to self and others.

Mind ____

____

Body ____

____

Spirit ____

____

Relationships____

____

Family ____

____

Business____

____

School ____

____

Career ____

____

Date / /

Power thought/quote: ____

What are you thankful for today? _____________________________________

____

____

Quiet time 5-10 minutes: Listen, read, meditate, write daily goals

____

____

____

Exercise: choose any activity you enjoy that will increase your heart rate to a point where you can answer a question but not carry on a conversation. Average 30 minutes. ____

Breakfast: ____
Snack:____
lunch: ____
Snack:____
Dinner: ____

Quiet time: Before bed take 15 minutes to reflect on the day. How did you do? Be kind and forgiving to self and others.

Mind ____

____

Body ____

____

Spirit ____

____

Relationships____

____

Family ____

____

Business____

____

School ____

____

Career ____

____

Date / /

Power thought/quote: ____

What are you thankful for today? _______________________________

____

____

Quiet time 5-10 minutes: Listen, read, meditate, write daily goals

____

____

____

Exercise: choose any activity you enjoy that will increase your heart rate to a point where you can answer a question but not carry on a conversation. Average 30 minutes. ____

Breakfast: ____
Snack:____
lunch: ____
Snack:____
Dinner: ____

Quiet time: Before bed take 15 minutes to reflect on the day. How did you do? Be kind and forgiving to self and others.

Mind ____

____

Body ____

____

Spirit ____

____

Relationships____

____

Family ____

____

Business____

____

School ____

____

Career ____

____

Date / /

Power thought/quote: _______________________________________

What are you thankful for today? _______________________________

____

____

Quiet time 5-10 minutes: Listen, read, meditate, write daily goals

____

____

____

Exercise: choose any activity you enjoy that will increase your heart rate to a point where you can answer a question but not carry on a conversation. Average 30 minutes. ____

Breakfast: ____

Snack:____

lunch: ____

Snack:____

Dinner: ____

Quiet time: Before bed take 15 minutes to reflect on the day. How did you do? Be kind and forgiving to self and others.

Mind ____

____

Body ____

____

Spirit ____

____

Relationships____

____

Family ____

____

Business____

____

School ____

____

Career ____

____

Date / /

Power thought/quote: ____

What are you thankful for today? ______________________________________
____
____

Quiet time 5-10 minutes: Listen, read, meditate, write daily goals
____
____
____

Exercise: choose any activity you enjoy that will increase your heart rate to a point where you can answer a question but not carry on a conversation. Average 30 minutes. ____

Breakfast: ____
Snack:____
lunch: ____
Snack:____
Dinner: ____

Quiet time: Before bed take 15 minutes to reflect on the day. How did you do? Be kind and forgiving to self and others.

Mind ____
____

Body____
____

Spirit ____
____

Relationships____
____

Family ____
____

Business____
____

School ____
____

Career ____
____

Date / /

Power thought/quote: _______________________________________

What are you thankful for today? _______________________________

____

____

Quiet time 5-10 minutes: Listen, read, meditate, write daily goals

____

____

____

Exercise: choose any activity you enjoy that will increase your heart rate to a point where you can answer a question but not carry on a conversation. Average 30 minutes. ____

Breakfast: ____

Snack:____

lunch: ____

Snack:____

Dinner: ____

Quiet time: Before bed take 15 minutes to reflect on the day. How did you do? Be kind and forgiving to self and others.

Mind ____

____

Body ____

____

Spirit ____

____

Relationships____

____

Family ____

____

Business____

____

School ____

____

Career ____

____

Date / /

Power thought/quote: ___________________________________

What are you thankful for today? _______________________

____

____

Quiet time 5-10 minutes: Listen, read, meditate, write daily goals

____

____

____

Exercise: choose any activity you enjoy that will increase your heart rate to a point where you can answer a question but not carry on a conversation. Average 30 minutes. ______________________________________

Breakfast: ____

Snack:____

lunch: ____

Snack:____

Dinner: ____

Quiet time: Before bed take 15 minutes to reflect on the day. How did you do? Be kind and forgiving to self and others.

Mind ____

____

Body ____

____

Spirit ____

____

Relationships____

____

Family ____

____

Business____

____

School ____

____

Career ____

____

Date / /

Power thought/quote: _______________________________________

What are you thankful for today? _______________________________
____
____

Quiet time 5-10 minutes: Listen, read, meditate, write daily goals

____
____
____

Exercise: choose any activity you enjoy that will increase your heart rate to a point where you can answer a question but not carry on a conversation. Average 30 minutes. ____

Breakfast: ____
Snack:____
lunch: ____
Snack:____
Dinner: ____

Quiet time: Before bed take 15 minutes to reflect on the day. How did you do? Be kind and forgiving to self and others.

Mind ____
____

Body ____
____

Spirit ____
____

Relationships____
____

Family ____
____

Business____
____

School ____
____

Career ____
____

Date / /

Power thought/quote: ____

What are you thankful for today? _______________________________

____

Quiet time 5-10 minutes: Listen, read, meditate, write daily goals

____

____

Exercise: choose any activity you enjoy that will increase your heart rate to a point where you can answer a question but not carry on a conversation. Average 30 minutes. ____

Breakfast: ____

Snack:____

lunch: ____

Snack:____

Dinner: ____

Quiet time: Before bed take 15 minutes to reflect on the day. How did you do? Be kind and forgiving to self and others.

Mind ____

Body ____

Spirit ____

Relationships ____

Family ____

Business____

School ____

Career ____

Date / /

Power thought/quote: _______________________________________

What are you thankful for today? _____________________________
____
____

Quiet time 5-10 minutes: Listen, read, meditate, write daily goals
____
____
____

Exercise: choose any activity you enjoy that will increase your heart rate to a point where you can answer a question but not carry on a conversation. Average 30 minutes. ____

Breakfast: ____
Snack:____
lunch: ____
Snack:____
Dinner: ____

Quiet time: Before bed take 15 minutes to reflect on the day. How did you do? Be kind and forgiving to self and others.

Mind ____
____

Body ____
____

Spirit ____
____

Relationships ____
____

Family ____
____

Business____
____

School ____
____

Career ____
____

Date / /

Power thought/quote: ___________________________

What are you thankful for today? ___________________________

____

____

Quiet time 5-10 minutes: Listen, read, meditate, write daily goals

____

____

____

Exercise: choose any activity you enjoy that will increase your heart rate to a point where you can answer a question but not carry on a conversation. Average 30 minutes. ___________________________

Breakfast: ___________________________
Snack:___________________________
lunch: ___________________________
Snack:___________________________
Dinner: ___________________________

Quiet time: Before bed take 15 minutes to reflect on the day. How did you do? Be kind and forgiving to self and others.

Mind ___________________________

Body ___________________________

Spirit ___________________________

Relationships ___________________________

Family ___________________________

Business___________________________

School ___________________________

Career ___________________________

Date / /

Power thought/quote: _______________________________________

What are you thankful for today? _____________________________

____

____

Quiet time 5-10 minutes: Listen, read, meditate, write daily goals

____

____

____

Exercise: choose any activity you enjoy that will increase your heart rate to a point where you can answer a question but not carry on a conversation. Average 30 minutes. ____

Breakfast: ____

Snack:____

lunch: ____

Snack:____

Dinner: ____

Quiet time: Before bed take 15 minutes to reflect on the day. How did you do? Be kind and forgiving to self and others.

Mind ____

____

Body ____

____

Spirit ____

____

Relationships ____

____

Family ____

____

Business____

____

School ____

____

Career ____

____

Date / /

Power thought/quote: _______________________________________

What are you thankful for today? _______________________________

____

____

Quiet time 5-10 minutes: Listen, read, meditate, write daily goals

____

____

____

Exercise: choose any activity you enjoy that will increase your heart rate to a point where you can answer a question but not carry on a conversation. Average 30 minutes. _______________________________

Breakfast: ____

Snack:____

lunch: ____

Snack:____

Dinner: ____

Quiet time: Before bed take 15 minutes to reflect on the day. How did you do? Be kind and forgiving to self and others.

Mind ____

____

Body ____

____

Spirit ____

____

Relationships ____

____

Family ____

____

Business____

____

School ____

____

Career ____

____

Date //

Power thought/quote: ____

What are you thankful for today? _______________________________________

____

____

Quiet time 5-10 minutes: Listen, read, meditate, write daily goals

____

____

____

Exercise: choose any activity you enjoy that will increase your heart rate to a point where you can answer a question but not carry on a conversation. Average 30 minutes. ____

Breakfast: ____

Snack:____

lunch: ____

Snack:____

Dinner: ____

Quiet time: Before bed take 15 minutes to reflect on the day. How did you do? Be kind and forgiving to self and others.

Mind ____

____

Body ____

____

Spirit ____

____

Relationships ____

____

Family ____

____

Business____

____

School ____

____

Career ____

____

Date / /

Power thought/quote: _______________________________

What are you thankful for today? _______________________________

____

____

Quiet time 5-10 minutes: Listen, read, meditate, write daily goals

____

____

____

Exercise: choose any activity you enjoy that will increase your heart rate to a point where you can answer a question but not carry on a conversation. Average 30 minutes. _______________________________

Breakfast: _______________________________
Snack:_______________________________
lunch: _______________________________
Snack:_______________________________
Dinner: _______________________________

Quiet time: Before bed take 15 minutes to reflect on the day. How did you do? Be kind and forgiving to self and others.

Mind _______________________________

____

Body _______________________________

____

Spirit _______________________________

____

Relationships _______________________________

____

Family _______________________________

____

Business_______________________________

____

School _______________________________

____

Career _______________________________

____

Date / /

Power thought/quote: _______________________________________

What are you thankful for today? ________________________________
____
____

Quiet time 5-10 minutes: Listen, read, meditate, write daily goals
____
____
____

Exercise: choose any activity you enjoy that will increase your heart rate to a point where you can answer a question but not carry on a conversation. Average 30 minutes. _______________________________________

Breakfast: ____
Snack:____
lunch: ____
Snack:____
Dinner: ____

Quiet time: Before bed take 15 minutes to reflect on the day. How did you do? Be kind and forgiving to self and others.

Mind ____
____

Body ____
____

Spirit ____
____

Relationships ____
____

Family ____
____

Business____
____

School ____
____

Career ____
____

Date / /

Power thought/quote: _______________________________________

What are you thankful for today? _____________________________

____

____

Quiet time 5-10 minutes: Listen, read, meditate, write daily goals

____

____

____

Exercise: choose any activity you enjoy that will increase your heart rate to a point where you can answer a question but not carry on a conversation. Average 30 minutes. ______________________________________

Breakfast: ____

Snack:____

lunch: ____

Snack:____

Dinner: ____

Quiet time: Before bed take 15 minutes to reflect on the day. How did you do? Be kind and forgiving to self and others.

Mind ____

____

Body ____

____

Spirit ____

____

Relationships ____

____

Family ____

____

Business____

____

School ____

____

Career ____

____

Date / /

Power thought/quote: _______________________________________

What are you thankful for today? ____________________________

____

____

Quiet time 5-10 minutes: Listen, read, meditate, write daily goals

____

____

____

Exercise: choose any activity you enjoy that will increase your heart rate to a point where you can answer a question but not carry on a conversation. Average 30 minutes. _______________________________________

Breakfast: ____

Snack:____

lunch: ____

Snack:____

Dinner: ____

Quiet time: Before bed take 15 minutes to reflect on the day. How did you do? Be kind and forgiving to self and others.

Mind ____

____

Body ____

____

Spirit ____

____

Relationships ____

____

Family ____

____

Business____

____

School ____

____

Career ____

____

Date / /

Power thought/quote: _______________________________________

What are you thankful for today? _______________________________

____

____

Quiet time 5-10 minutes: Listen, read, meditate, write daily goals

____

____

____

Exercise: choose any activity you enjoy that will increase your heart rate to a point where you can answer a question but not carry on a conversation. Average 30 minutes. ____

Breakfast: ____

Snack:____

lunch: ____

Snack:____

Dinner: ____

Quiet time: Before bed take 15 minutes to reflect on the day. How did you do? Be kind and forgiving to self and others.

Mind ____

____

Body ____

____

Spirit ____

____

Relationships ____

____

Family ____

____

Business____

____

School ____

____

Career ____

____

Date / /

Power thought/quote: _______________________________________

What are you thankful for today? _____________________________
____
____

Quiet time 5-10 minutes: Listen, read, meditate, write daily goals
____
____
____

Exercise: choose any activity you enjoy that will increase your heart rate to a point where you can answer a question but not carry on a conversation. Average 30 minutes. ____

Breakfast: ____
Snack:____
lunch: ____
Snack:____
Dinner: ____

Quiet time: Before bed take 15 minutes to reflect on the day. How did you do? Be kind and forgiving to self and others.

Mind ____
____

Body ____
____

Spirit ____
____

Relationships ____
____

Family ____
____

Business____
____

School ____
____

Career ____
____

Date / /

Power thought/quote: _______________________________

What are you thankful for today? _____________________
____
____

Quiet time 5-10 minutes: Listen, read, meditate, write daily goals
____
____
____

Exercise: choose any activity you enjoy that will increase your heart rate to a point where you can answer a question but not carry on a conversation. Average 30 minutes. _______________________________________

Breakfast: ____
Snack:____
lunch: ____
Snack:____
Dinner: ____

Quiet time: Before bed take 15 minutes to reflect on the day. How did you do? Be kind and forgiving to self and others.

Mind ____
____

Body ____
____

Spirit ____
____

Relationships ____
____

Family ____
____

Business____
____

School ____
____

Career ____
____

Date / /

Power thought/quote: _______________________________________

What are you thankful for today? ________________________________

____

____

Quiet time 5-10 minutes: Listen, read, meditate, write daily goals

____

____

____

Exercise: choose any activity you enjoy that will increase your heart rate to a point where you can answer a question but not carry on a conversation. Average 30 minutes. ____

Breakfast: ____

Snack:____

lunch: ____

Snack:____

Dinner: ____

Quiet time: Before bed take 15 minutes to reflect on the day. How did you do? Be kind and forgiving to self and others.

Mind ____

____

Body ____

____

Spirit ____

____

Relationships ____

____

Family ____

____

Business____

____

School ____

____

Career ____

____

Date / /

Power thought/quote: _______________________________

What are you thankful for today? _______________________________
____
____

Quiet time 5-10 minutes: Listen, read, meditate, write daily goals
____
____
____

Exercise: choose any activity you enjoy that will increase your heart rate to a point where you can answer a question but not carry on a conversation. Average 30 minutes. _______________________________

Breakfast: _______________________________
Snack:_______________________________
lunch: _______________________________
Snack:_______________________________
Dinner: _______________________________

Quiet time: Before bed take 15 minutes to reflect on the day. How did you do? Be kind and forgiving to self and others.

Mind _______________________________
____

Body _______________________________
____

Spirit _______________________________
____

Relationships _______________________________
____

Family _______________________________
____

Business_______________________________
____

School _______________________________
____

Career _______________________________
____

Date / /

Power thought/quote: ____

What are you thankful for today? ______________________________________
____
____

Quiet time 5-10 minutes: Listen, read, meditate, write daily goals

____
____
____

Exercise: choose any activity you enjoy that will increase your heart rate to a point where you can answer a question but not carry on a conversation. Average 30 minutes. ____

Breakfast: ____
Snack:____
lunch: ____
Snack:____
Dinner: ____

Quiet time: Before bed take 15 minutes to reflect on the day. How did you do? Be kind and forgiving to self and others.

Mind ____
____

Body ____
____

Spirit ____
____

Relationships ____
____

Family ____
____

Business____
____

School ____
____

Career ____
____

Date / /

Power thought/quote: ____

What are you thankful for today? ______________________________

____

____

Quiet time 5-10 minutes: Listen, read, meditate, write daily goals

____

____

____

Exercise: choose any activity you enjoy that will increase your heart rate to a point where you can answer a question but not carry on a conversation. Average 30 minutes. ____

Breakfast: ____

Snack:____

lunch: ____

Snack:____

Dinner: ____

Quiet time: Before bed take 15 minutes to reflect on the day. How did you do? Be kind and forgiving to self and others.

Mind ____

____

Body ____

____

Spirit ____

____

Relationships ____

____

Family ____

____

Business____

____

School ____

____

Career ____

____

Date / /

Power thought/quote: _______________________________________

What are you thankful for today? _______________________________

____

____

Quiet time 5-10 minutes: Listen, read, meditate, write daily goals

____

____

____

Exercise: choose any activity you enjoy that will increase your heart rate to a point where you can answer a question but not carry on a conversation. Average 30 minutes. _______________________________________

Breakfast: ____

Snack: ____

lunch: ____

Snack: ____

Dinner: ____

Quiet time: Before bed take 15 minutes to reflect on the day. How did you do? Be kind and forgiving to self and others.

Mind ____

____

Body ____

____

Spirit ____

____

Relationships ____

____

Family ____

____

Business ____

____

School ____

____

Career ____

____

Date / /

Power thought/quote: _______________________________________

What are you thankful for today? _______________________________
____
____

Quiet time 5-10 minutes: Listen, read, meditate, write daily goals
____
____
____

Exercise: choose any activity you enjoy that will increase your heart rate to a point where you can answer a question but not carry on a conversation. Average 30 minutes. ____

Breakfast: ____
Snack:____
lunch: ____
Snack:____
Dinner: ____

Quiet time: Before bed take 15 minutes to reflect on the day. How did you do? Be kind and forgiving to self and others.

Mind ____
____

Body ____
____

Spirit ____
____

Relationships ____
____

Family ____
____

Business____
____

School ____
____

Career ____
____

Date / /

Power thought/quote: _________________________________

What are you thankful for today? _________________________

____

____

Quiet time 5-10 minutes: Listen, read, meditate, write daily goals

____

____

____

Exercise: choose any activity you enjoy that will increase your heart rate to a point where you can answer a question but not carry on a conversation. Average 30 minutes. ____

Breakfast: ____

Snack:____

lunch: ____

Snack:____

Dinner: ____

Quiet time: Before bed take 15 minutes to reflect on the day. How did you do? Be kind and forgiving to self and others.

Mind ____

____

Body ____

____

Spirit ____

____

Relationships ____

____

Family ____

____

Business____

____

School ____

____

Career ____

____

Date / /

Power thought/quote: ____________________________________

What are you thankful for today? ____________________________
____
____

Quiet time 5-10 minutes: Listen, read, meditate, write daily goals
____
____
____

Exercise: choose any activity you enjoy that will increase your heart rate to a point where you can answer a question but not carry on a conversation. Average 30 minutes. ____________________________________

Breakfast: ____
Snack:____
lunch: ____
Snack:____
Dinner: ____

Quiet time: Before bed take 15 minutes to reflect on the day. How did you do? Be kind and forgiving to self and others.

Mind ____
____

Body ____
____

Spirit ____
____

Relationships ____
____

Family ____
____

Business____
____

School ____
____

Career ____
____

Date / /

Power thought/quote: ____

What are you thankful for today? _______________________________________

____

____

Quiet time 5-10 minutes: Listen, read, meditate, write daily goals

____

____

____

Exercise: choose any activity you enjoy that will increase your heart rate to a point where you can answer a question but not carry on a conversation. Average 30 minutes. ____

Breakfast: ____

Snack:____

lunch: ____

Snack:____

Dinner: ____

Quiet time: Before bed take 15 minutes to reflect on the day. How did you do? Be kind and forgiving to self and others.

Mind ____

____

Body ____

____

Spirit ____

____

Relationships ____

____

Family ____

____

Business____

____

School ____

____

Career ____

____

Date / /

Power thought/quote: ____________________________________

What are you thankful for today? ____________________________

____

____

Quiet time 5-10 minutes: Listen, read, meditate, write daily goals

____

____

____

Exercise: choose any activity you enjoy that will increase your heart rate to a point where you can answer a question but not carry on a conversation. Average 30 minutes. __________________________________

Breakfast: ____

Snack:____

lunch: ____

Snack:____

Dinner: ____

Quiet time: Before bed take 15 minutes to reflect on the day. How did you do? Be kind and forgiving to self and others.

Mind ____

____

Body ____

____

Spirit ____

____

Relationships ____

____

Family ____

____

Business____

____

School ____

____

Career ____

____

Date / /

Power thought/quote: ____

What are you thankful for today? ______________________________________
____
____

Quiet time 5-10 minutes: Listen, read, meditate, write daily goals
____
____
____

Exercise: choose any activity you enjoy that will increase your heart rate to a point where you can answer a question but not carry on a conversation. Average 30 minutes. ____

Breakfast: ____
Snack:____
lunch: ____
Snack:____
Dinner: ____

Quiet time: Before bed take 15 minutes to reflect on the day. How did you do? Be kind and forgiving to self and others.

Mind ____
____

Body ____
____

Spirit ____
____

Relationships ____
____

Family ____
____

Business____
____

School ____
____

Career ____
____

Date / /

Power thought/quote: _______________________________

What are you thankful for today? _______________________
____
____

Quiet time 5-10 minutes: Listen, read, meditate, write daily goals
____
____
____

Exercise: choose any activity you enjoy that will increase your heart rate to a point where you can answer a question but not carry on a conversation. Average 30 minutes. ______________________________________

Breakfast: ____
Snack:____
lunch: ____
Snack:____
Dinner: ____

Quiet time: Before bed take 15 minutes to reflect on the day. How did you do? Be kind and forgiving to self and others.

Mind ____
____
Body ____
____
Spirit ____
____
Relationships ____
____
Family ____
____
Business____
____
School ____
____
Career ____
____

Date / /

Power thought/quote: ____

What are you thankful for today? _______________________________________
____
____

Quiet time 5-10 minutes: Listen, read, meditate, write daily goals
____
____
____

Exercise: choose any activity you enjoy that will increase your heart rate to a point where you can answer a question but not carry on a conversation. Average 30 minutes. ____

Breakfast: ____
Snack:____
lunch: ____
Snack:____
Dinner: ____

Quiet time: Before bed take 15 minutes to reflect on the day. How did you do? Be kind and forgiving to self and others.

Mind ____
____

Body ____
____

Spirit ____
____

Relationships ____
____

Family ____
____

Business____
____

School ____
____

Career ____
____

Date / /

Power thought/quote: _______________________________________

What are you thankful for today? _______________________________

____

Quiet time 5-10 minutes: Listen, read, meditate, write daily goals

____

____

____

Exercise: choose any activity you enjoy that will increase your heart rate to a point where you can answer a question but not carry on a conversation. Average 30 minutes. ____

Breakfast: ____

Snack:____

lunch: ____

Snack:____

Dinner: ____

Quiet time: Before bed take 15 minutes to reflect on the day. How did you do? Be kind and forgiving to self and others.

Mind ____

____

Body ____

____

Spirit ____

____

Relationships ____

____

Family ____

____

Business____

____

School ____

____

Career ____

____

Date / /

Power thought/quote: _______________________________________

What are you thankful for today? _______________________________
____
____

Quiet time 5-10 minutes: Listen, read, meditate, write daily goals

____
____
____

Exercise: choose any activity you enjoy that will increase your heart rate to a point where you can answer a question but not carry on a conversation. Average 30 minutes. ____

Breakfast: ____
Snack:____
lunch: ____
Snack:____
Dinner: ____

Quiet time: Before bed take 15 minutes to reflect on the day. How did you do? Be kind and forgiving to self and others.

Mind ____
____

Body ____
____

Spirit ____
____

Relationships ____
____

Family ____
____

Business____
____

School ____
____

Career ____
____

Date / /

Power thought/quote: ____

What are you thankful for today? _______________________________

____

____

Quiet time 5-10 minutes: Listen, read, meditate, write daily goals

____

____

____

Exercise: choose any activity you enjoy that will increase your heart rate to a point where you can answer a question but not carry on a conversation. Average 30 minutes. _______________________________

Breakfast: ____
Snack:____
lunch: ____
Snack:____
Dinner: ____

Quiet time: Before bed take 15 minutes to reflect on the day. How did you do? Be kind and forgiving to self and others.

Mind ____

____

Body ____

____

Spirit ____

____

Relationships ____

____

Family ____

____

Business____

____

School ____

____

Career ____

____

Date / /

Power thought/quote: ____

What are you thankful for today? _______________________________________

____

____

Quiet time 5-10 minutes: Listen, read, meditate, write daily goals

____

____

____

Exercise: choose any activity you enjoy that will increase your heart rate to a point where you can answer a question but not carry on a conversation. Average 30 minutes. ____

Breakfast: ____

Snack:____

lunch: ____

Snack:____

Dinner: ____

Quiet time: Before bed take 15 minutes to reflect on the day. How did you do? Be kind and forgiving to self and others.

Mind ____

____

Body ____

____

Spirit ____

____

Relationships ____

____

Family ____

____

Business____

____

School ____

____

Career ____

____

Date / /

Power thought/quote: _______________________________

What are you thankful for today? _______________________

____

Quiet time 5-10 minutes: Listen, read, meditate, write daily goals

____

____

Exercise: choose any activity you enjoy that will increase your heart rate to a point where you can answer a question but not carry on a conversation. Average 30 minutes. _______________________________

Breakfast: ____

Snack:____

lunch: ____

Snack:____

Dinner: ____

Quiet time: Before bed take 15 minutes to reflect on the day. How did you do? Be kind and forgiving to self and others.

Mind ____

____

Body ____

____

Spirit ____

____

Relationships ____

____

Family ____

____

Business____

____

School ____

____

Career ____

____

Date / /

Power thought/quote: _______________________________________

What are you thankful for today? _______________________________
____
____

Quiet time 5-10 minutes: Listen, read, meditate, write daily goals
____
____
____

Exercise: choose any activity you enjoy that will increase your heart rate to a point where you can answer a question but not carry on a conversation. Average 30 minutes. ____

Breakfast: ____
Snack:____
lunch: ____
Snack:____
Dinner: ____

Quiet time: Before bed take 15 minutes to reflect on the day. How did you do? Be kind and forgiving to self and others.

Mind ____
____

Body ____
____

Spirit ____
____

Relationships ____
____

Family ____
____

Business____
____

School ____
____

Career ____
____

Date / /

Power thought/quote: ___________________________________

What are you thankful for today? _________________________
____
____

Quiet time 5-10 minutes: Listen, read, meditate, write daily goals
____
____
____

Exercise: choose any activity you enjoy that will increase your heart rate to a point where you can answer a question but not carry on a conversation. Average 30 minutes. _______________________________

Breakfast: ____
Snack:____
lunch: ____
Snack:____
Dinner: ____

Quiet time: Before bed take 15 minutes to reflect on the day. How did you do? Be kind and forgiving to self and others.

Mind ____
____

Body ____
____

Spirit ____
____

Relationships ____
____

Family ____
____

Business____
____

School ____
____

Career ____
____

Date / /

Power thought/quote: ____

What are you thankful for today? _______________________________________

____

____

Quiet time 5-10 minutes: Listen, read, meditate, write daily goals

____

____

____

Exercise: choose any activity you enjoy that will increase your heart rate to a point where you can answer a question but not carry on a conversation. Average 30 minutes. ____

Breakfast: ____
Snack:____
lunch: ____
Snack:____
Dinner: ____

Quiet time: Before bed take 15 minutes to reflect on the day. How did you do? Be kind and forgiving to self and others.

Mind ____

____

Body ____

____

Spirit ____

____

Relationships ____

____

Family ____

____

Business____

____

School ____

____

Career ____

____

Date / /

Power thought/quote: _______________________________________

What are you thankful for today? _______________________________

____

____

Quiet time 5-10 minutes: Listen, read, meditate, write daily goals

____

____

____

Exercise: choose any activity you enjoy that will increase your heart rate to a point where you can answer a question but not carry on a conversation. Average 30 minutes. _______________________________________

Breakfast: ____
Snack:____
lunch: ____
Snack:____
Dinner: ____

Quiet time: Before bed take 15 minutes to reflect on the day. How did you do? Be kind and forgiving to self and others.

Mind ____

____

Body ____

____

Spirit ____

____

Relationships ____

____

Family ____

____

Business____

____

School ____

____

Career ____

____

Date / /

Power thought/quote: _______________________________________

What are you thankful for today? _____________________________

____

____

Quiet time 5-10 minutes: Listen, read, meditate, write daily goals

____

____

____

Exercise: choose any activity you enjoy that will increase your heart rate to a point where you can answer a question but not carry on a conversation. Average 30 minutes. ____

Breakfast: ____

Snack:____

lunch: ____

Snack:____

Dinner: ____

Quiet time: Before bed take 15 minutes to reflect on the day. How did you do? Be kind and forgiving to self and others.

Mind ____

____

Body ____

____

Spirit ____

____

Relationships ____

____

Family ____

____

Business____

____

School ____

____

Career ____

____

Date / /

Power thought/quote: _______________________________________

What are you thankful for today? ______________________________

____

Quiet time 5-10 minutes: Listen, read, meditate, write daily goals

____

____

____

Exercise: choose any activity you enjoy that will increase your heart rate to a point where you can answer a question but not carry on a conversation. Average 30 minutes. ____

Breakfast: ____

Snack:____

lunch: ____

Snack:____

Dinner: ____

Quiet time: Before bed take 15 minutes to reflect on the day. How did you do? Be kind and forgiving to self and others.

Mind ____

____

Body ____

____

Spirit ____

____

Relationships ____

____

Family ____

____

Business____

____

School ____

____

Career ____

____

Date / /

Power thought/quote: _______________________________________

What are you thankful for today? _______________________________
____
____

Quiet time 5-10 minutes: Listen, read, meditate, write daily goals
____
____
____

Exercise: choose any activity you enjoy that will increase your heart rate to a point where you can answer a question but not carry on a conversation. Average 30 minutes. _______________________________________

Breakfast: ____
Snack:____
lunch: ____
Snack:____
Dinner: ____

Quiet time: Before bed take 15 minutes to reflect on the day. How did you do? Be kind and forgiving to self and others.

Mind ____
____

Body ____
____

Spirit ____
____

Relationships ____
____

Family ____
____

Business____
____

School ____
____

Career ____
____

Date / /

Power thought/quote: _______________________________________

What are you thankful for today? _______________________________
____
____

Quiet time 5-10 minutes: Listen, read, meditate, write daily goals
____
____
____

Exercise: choose any activity you enjoy that will increase your heart rate to a point where you can answer a question but not carry on a conversation. Average 30 minutes. _______________________________________

Breakfast: ____
Snack:____
lunch: ____
Snack:____
Dinner: ____

Quiet time: Before bed take 15 minutes to reflect on the day. How did you do? Be kind and forgiving to self and others.

Mind ____
____

Body ____
____

Spirit ____
____

Relationships ____
____

Family ____
____

Business____
____

School ____
____

Career ____
____

Date / /

Power thought/quote: ____

What are you thankful for today? _______________________________________

____

____

Quiet time 5-10 minutes: Listen, read, meditate, write daily goals

____

____

____

Exercise: choose any activity you enjoy that will increase your heart rate to a point where you can answer a question but not carry on a conversation. Average 30 minutes. ____

Breakfast: ____

Snack:____

lunch: ____

Snack:____

Dinner: ____

Quiet time: Before bed take 15 minutes to reflect on the day. How did you do? Be kind and forgiving to self and others.

Mind ____

____

Body ____

____

Spirit ____

____

Relationships ____

____

Family ____

____

Business____

____

School ____

____

Career ____

____

Date / /

Power thought/quote: ___________________________

What are you thankful for today? ___________________________

____

____

Quiet time 5-10 minutes: Listen, read, meditate, write daily goals

____

____

____

Exercise: choose any activity you enjoy that will increase your heart rate to a point where you can answer a question but not carry on a conversation. Average 30 minutes. ___________________________

Breakfast: ___________________________
Snack:___________________________
lunch: ___________________________
Snack:___________________________
Dinner: ___________________________

Quiet time: Before bed take 15 minutes to reflect on the day. How did you do? Be kind and forgiving to self and others.

Mind ___________________________

____

Body ___________________________

____

Spirit ___________________________

____

Relationships ___________________________

____

Family ___________________________

____

Business___________________________

____

School ___________________________

____

Career ___________________________

____

Date / /

Power thought/quote: ____

What are you thankful for today? _______________________________________

____

____

Quiet time 5-10 minutes: Listen, read, meditate, write daily goals

____

____

____

Exercise: choose any activity you enjoy that will increase your heart rate to a point where you can answer a question but not carry on a conversation. Average 30 minutes. ____

Breakfast: ____

Snack:____

lunch: ____

Snack:____

Dinner: ____

Quiet time: Before bed take 15 minutes to reflect on the day. How did you do? Be kind and forgiving to self and others.

Mind ____

____

Body ____

____

Spirit ____

____

Relationships ____

____

Family ____

____

Business____

____

School ____

____

Career ____

____

Date / /

Power thought/quote: ________________________________

What are you thankful for today? ________________________________
____
____

Quiet time 5-10 minutes: Listen, read, meditate, write daily goals

____
____
____

Exercise: choose any activity you enjoy that will increase your heart rate to a point where you can answer a question but not carry on a conversation. Average 30 minutes. ________________________________

Breakfast: ________________________________
Snack:________________________________
lunch: ________________________________
Snack:________________________________
Dinner: ________________________________

Quiet time: Before bed take 15 minutes to reflect on the day. How did you do? Be kind and forgiving to self and others.

Mind ________________________________
____

Body ________________________________
____

Spirit ________________________________
____

Relationships ________________________________
____

Family ________________________________
____

Business________________________________
____

School ________________________________
____

Career ________________________________
____

Date / /

Power thought/quote: ___________________________________

What are you thankful for today? ___________________________

____

____

Quiet time 5-10 minutes: Listen, read, meditate, write daily goals

____

____

____

Exercise: choose any activity you enjoy that will increase your heart rate to a point where you can answer a question but not carry on a conversation. Average 30 minutes. ____

Breakfast: ____

Snack:____

lunch: ____

Snack:____

Dinner: ____

Quiet time: Before bed take 15 minutes to reflect on the day. How did you do? Be kind and forgiving to self and others.

Mind ____

____

Body ____

____

Spirit ____

____

Relationships ____

____

Family ____

____

Business____

____

School ____

____

Career ____

____

Date / /

Power thought/quote: ____

What are you thankful for today? _____________________________________

____

____

Quiet time 5-10 minutes: Listen, read, meditate, write daily goals

____

____

____

Exercise: choose any activity you enjoy that will increase your heart rate to a point where you can answer a question but not carry on a conversation. Average 30 minutes. ____

Breakfast: ____
Snack:____
lunch: ____
Snack:____
Dinner: ____

Quiet time: Before bed take 15 minutes to reflect on the day. How did you do? Be kind and forgiving to self and others.

Mind ____

____

Body ____

____

Spirit ____

____

Relationships____

____

Family ____

____

Business____

____

School ____

____

Career ____

____

Date / /

Power thought/quote: _______________________________

What are you thankful for today? _______________________

____

____

Quiet time 5-10 minutes: Listen, read, meditate, write daily goals

____

____

____

Exercise: choose any activity you enjoy that will increase your heart rate to a point where you can answer a question but not carry on a conversation. Average 30 minutes. _______________________________

Breakfast: _______________________________

Snack:_______________________________

lunch: _______________________________

Snack:_______________________________

Dinner: _______________________________

Quiet time: Before bed take 15 minutes to reflect on the day. How did you do? Be kind and forgiving to self and others.

Mind _______________________________

____

Body _______________________________

____

Spirit _______________________________

____

Relationships _______________________________

____

Family _______________________________

____

Business_______________________________

____

School _______________________________

____

Career _______________________________

____

Date / /

Power thought/quote: _______________________________________

What are you thankful for today? _______________________________

____

Quiet time 5-10 minutes: Listen, read, meditate, write daily goals

____

____

____

Exercise: choose any activity you enjoy that will increase your heart rate to a point where you can answer a question but not carry on a conversation. Average 30 minutes. _______________________________________

Breakfast: ____

Snack:____

lunch: ____

Snack:____

Dinner: ____

Quiet time: Before bed take 15 minutes to reflect on the day. How did you do? Be kind and forgiving to self and others.

Mind ____

____

Body ____

____

Spirit ____

____

Relationships ____

____

Family ____

____

Business____

____

School____

____

Career ____

____

Date / /

Power thought/quote: ____

What are you thankful for today? _______________________________
____
____

Quiet time 5-10 minutes: Listen, read, meditate, write daily goals
____
____
____

Exercise: choose any activity you enjoy that will increase your heart rate to a point where you can answer a question but not carry on a conversation. Average 30 minutes. ____

Breakfast: ____
Snack:____
lunch: ____
Snack:____
Dinner: ____

Quiet time: Before bed take 15 minutes to reflect on the day. How did you do? Be kind and forgiving to self and others.

Mind ____
____

Body ____
____

Spirit ____
____

Relationships ____
____

Family ____
____

Business____
____

School ____
____

Career ____
____

Date / /

Power thought/quote: _______________________________________

What are you thankful for today? _____________________________
____
____

Quiet time 5-10 minutes: Listen, read, meditate, write daily goals
____
____
____

Exercise: choose any activity you enjoy that will increase your heart rate to a point where you can answer a question but not carry on a conversation. Average 30 minutes. _______________________________________

Breakfast: ____
Snack:____
lunch: ____
Snack:____
Dinner: ____

Quiet time: Before bed take 15 minutes to reflect on the day. How did you do? Be kind and forgiving to self and others.

Mind ____
____

Body ____
____

Spirit ____
____

Relationships ____
____

Family ____
____

Business____
____

School ____
____

Career ____
____

Date / /

Power thought/quote: _______________________________________

What are you thankful for today? _______________________________
____
____

Quiet time 5-10 minutes: Listen, read, meditate, write daily goals
____
____
____

Exercise: choose any activity you enjoy that will increase your heart rate to a point where you can answer a question but not carry on a conversation. Average 30 minutes. ____

Breakfast: ____
Snack:____
lunch: ____
Snack:____
Dinner: ____

Quiet time: Before bed take 15 minutes to reflect on the day. How did you do? Be kind and forgiving to self and others.

Mind ____
____

Body ____
____

Spirit ____
____

Relationships ____
____

Family ____
____

Business____
____

School ____
____

Career ____
____

Date / /

Power thought/quote: _______________________________________

What are you thankful for today? _______________________________
____
____

Quiet time 5-10 minutes: Listen, read, meditate, write daily goals
____
____
____

Exercise: choose any activity you enjoy that will increase your heart rate to a point where you can answer a question but not carry on a conversation. Average 30 minutes. _______________________________________

Breakfast: ____
Snack:____
lunch: ____
Snack:____
Dinner: ____

Quiet time: Before bed take 15 minutes to reflect on the day. How did you do? Be kind and forgiving to self and others.

Mind ____
____

Body ____
____

Spirit ____
____

Relationships ____
____

Family ____
____

Business____
____

School ____
____

Career ____
____

Date / /

Power thought/quote: ____

What are you thankful for today? _______________________________________

____

____

Quiet time 5-10 minutes: Listen, read, meditate, write daily goals

____

____

____

Exercise: choose any activity you enjoy that will increase your heart rate to a point where you can answer a question but not carry on a conversation. Average 30 minutes. ____

Breakfast: ____

Snack:____

lunch: ____

Snack:____

Dinner: ____

Quiet time: Before bed take 15 minutes to reflect on the day. How did you do? Be kind and forgiving to self and others.

Mind ____

____

Body ____

____

Spirit ____

____

Relationships ____

____

Family ____

____

Business____

____

School ____

____

Career ____

____

Date / /

Power thought/quote: _______________________________________

What are you thankful for today? _____________________________

____

____

Quiet time 5-10 minutes: Listen, read, meditate, write daily goals

____

____

____

Exercise: choose any activity you enjoy that will increase your heart rate to a point where you can answer a question but not carry on a conversation. Average 30 minutes. _______________________________________

Breakfast: ____
Snack:____
lunch: ____
Snack:____
Dinner: ____

Quiet time: Before bed take 15 minutes to reflect on the day. How did you do? Be kind and forgiving to self and others.

Mind ____

____

Body ____

____

Spirit ____

____

Relationships ____

____

Family ____

____

Business____

____

School ____

____

Career ____

____

Date / /

Power thought/quote: ____

What are you thankful for today? ______________________________________
____
____

Quiet time 5-10 minutes: Listen, read, meditate, write daily goals

____
____
____

Exercise: choose any activity you enjoy that will increase your heart rate to a point where you can answer a question but not carry on a conversation. Average 30 minutes. ____

Breakfast: ____
Snack:____
lunch: ____
Snack:____
Dinner: ____

Quiet time: Before bed take 15 minutes to reflect on the day. How did you do? Be kind and forgiving to self and others.

Mind ____
____

Body ____
____

Spirit ____
____

Relationships ____
____

Family ____
____

Business____
____

School ____
____

Career ____
____

Date / /

Power thought/quote: _______________________________________

What are you thankful for today? _____________________________

____

____

Quiet time 5-10 minutes: Listen, read, meditate, write daily goals

____

____

____

Exercise: choose any activity you enjoy that will increase your heart rate to a point where you can answer a question but not carry on a conversation. Average 30 minutes. _______________________________________

Breakfast: ____

Snack:____

lunch: ____

Snack:____

Dinner: ____

Quiet time: Before bed take 15 minutes to reflect on the day. How did you do? Be kind and forgiving to self and others.

Mind ____

____

Body ____

____

Spirit ____

____

Relationships ____

____

Family ____

____

Business____

____

School ____

____

Career ____

____

Date / /

Power thought/quote: _______________________________________

What are you thankful for today? _______________________________
____
____

Quiet time 5-10 minutes: Listen, read, meditate, write daily goals
____
____
____

Exercise: choose any activity you enjoy that will increase your heart rate to a point where you can answer a question but not carry on a conversation. Average 30 minutes. ____

Breakfast: ____
Snack:____
lunch: ____
Snack:____
Dinner: ____

Quiet time: Before bed take 15 minutes to reflect on the day. How did you do? Be kind and forgiving to self and others.

Mind ____
____

Body ____
____

Spirit ____
____

Relationships ____
____

Family ____
____

Business____
____

School ____
____

Career ____
____

Date / /

Power thought/quote: _______________________________

What are you thankful for today? _______________________
____
____

Quiet time 5-10 minutes: Listen, read, meditate, write daily goals
____
____
____

Exercise: choose any activity you enjoy that will increase your heart rate to a point where you can answer a question but not carry on a conversation. Average 30 minutes. _______________________________________

Breakfast: _______________________________________
Snack:____
lunch: ____
Snack:____
Dinner: ____

Quiet time: Before bed take 15 minutes to reflect on the day. How did you do? Be kind and forgiving to self and others.

Mind _______________________________________
____

Body _______________________________________
____

Spirit _______________________________________
____

Relationships _______________________________________
____

Family _______________________________________
____

Business_______________________________________
____

School _______________________________________
____

Career _______________________________________
____

Date / /

Power thought/quote: _______________________________

What are you thankful for today? _______________________________

____

____

Quiet time 5-10 minutes: Listen, read, meditate, write daily goals

____

____

____

Exercise: choose any activity you enjoy that will increase your heart rate to a point where you can answer a question but not carry on a conversation. Average 30 minutes. _______________________________

Breakfast: _______________________________

Snack:_______________________________

lunch: _______________________________

Snack:_______________________________

Dinner: _______________________________

Quiet time: Before bed take 15 minutes to reflect on the day. How did you do? Be kind and forgiving to self and others.

Mind _______________________________

____

Body _______________________________

____

Spirit _______________________________

____

Relationships _______________________________

____

Family _______________________________

____

Business_______________________________

____

School _______________________________

____

Career _______________________________

____

Date / /

Power thought/quote: ____

What are you thankful for today? _______________________________

____

____

Quiet time 5-10 minutes: Listen, read, meditate, write daily goals

____

____

____

Exercise: choose any activity you enjoy that will increase your heart rate to a point where you can answer a question but not carry on a conversation. Average 30 minutes. _______________________________________

Breakfast: ____

Snack:____

lunch: ____

Snack:____

Dinner: ____

Quiet time: Before bed take 15 minutes to reflect on the day. How did you do? Be kind and forgiving to self and others.

Mind ____

____

Body ____

____

Spirit ____

____

Relationships ____

____

Family ____

____

Business____

____

School ____

____

Career ____

____

Date / /

Power thought/quote: ____

What are you thankful for today? _______________________________________
____
____

Quiet time 5-10 minutes: Listen, read, meditate, write daily goals
____
____
____

Exercise: choose any activity you enjoy that will increase your heart rate to a point where you can answer a question but not carry on a conversation. Average 30 minutes. ____

Breakfast: ____

Snack:____

lunch: ____

Snack:____

Dinner: ____

Quiet time: Before bed take 15 minutes to reflect on the day. How did you do? Be kind and forgiving to self and others.

Mind ____
____

Body ____
____

Spirit ____
____

Relationships ____
____

Family ____
____

Business____
____

School ____
____

Career ____
____

Date / /

Power thought/quote: _______________________________________

What are you thankful for today? _____________________________

____

____

Quiet time 5-10 minutes: Listen, read, meditate, write daily goals

____

____

____

Exercise: choose any activity you enjoy that will increase your heart rate to a point where you can answer a question but not carry on a conversation. Average 30 minutes. ____

Breakfast: ____

Snack:____

lunch: ____

Snack:____

Dinner: ____

Quiet time: Before bed take 15 minutes to reflect on the day. How did you do? Be kind and forgiving to self and others.

Mind ____

____

Body ____

____

Spirit ____

____

Relationships ____

____

Family ____

____

Business____

____

School ____

____

Career ____

____

Date / /

Power thought/quote: ____

What are you thankful for today? _______________________________________
____
____

Quiet time 5-10 minutes: Listen, read, meditate, write daily goals
____
____
____

Exercise: choose any activity you enjoy that will increase your heart rate to a point where you can answer a question but not carry on a conversation. Average 30 minutes. ____

Breakfast: ____
Snack:____
lunch: ____
Snack:____
Dinner: ____

Quiet time: Before bed take 15 minutes to reflect on the day. How did you do? Be kind and forgiving to self and others.

Mind ____
____

Body ____
____

Spirit ____
____

Relationships ____
____

Family ____
____

Business____
____

School ____
____

Career ____
____

Date / /

Power thought/quote: _______________________________________

What are you thankful for today? _____________________________

____

____

Quiet time 5-10 minutes: Listen, read, meditate, write daily goals

____

____

____

Exercise: choose any activity you enjoy that will increase your heart rate to a point where you can answer a question but not carry on a conversation. Average 30 minutes. ____

Breakfast: ____
Snack:____
lunch: ____
Snack:____
Dinner: ____

Quiet time: Before bed take 15 minutes to reflect on the day. How did you do? Be kind and forgiving to self and others.

Mind ____

____

Body ____

____

Spirit ____

____

Relationships ____

____

Family ____

____

Business____

____

School ____

____

Career ____

____

Date / /

Power thought/quote: _______________________________

What are you thankful for today? _______________________

____

____

Quiet time 5-10 minutes: Listen, read, meditate, write daily goals

____

____

____

Exercise: choose any activity you enjoy that will increase your heart rate to a point where you can answer a question but not carry on a conversation. Average 30 minutes. _______________________________________

Breakfast: _____________________________________

Snack:____

lunch: ____

Snack:____

Dinner: _______________________________________

Quiet time: Before bed take 15 minutes to reflect on the day. How did you do? Be kind and forgiving to self and others.

Mind ____

____

Body ____

____

Spirit ____

____

Relationships ___________________________________

____

Family ____

____

Business_______________________________________

____

School ____

____

Career ____

____

References

Burnaby, BC: (1997), 559 *The encyclopedia of Natural Healing,* Alive Publishing Group,

David C. Cook, *Quiet moments with God Devotional Journal (2003),* first edition, Honor Books, Colorado Springs, CO 80918 U.S.A

Dianne Hales, *An Invitation to health(2005),* seventh edition, Thompson Wadsworth, Baltimore, CA. U.S.A.

George Malkmus with Peter and Stow Shockey, *The Hallelujah Diet(2006)* Destiny Image Publishers, Inc., Shippenburg, PA 17257-0310 U.S.A.

Neil Nedley, M.D. *Proof Positive: How to Reliably Combat Disease and Achieve Optimal Health through Nutrition and Lifestyle (1999)* Quality Books Inc., NW, Ardmore, OK 73401 U.S.A.

New King James Version bible (1982) Thomas Nelson, Inc.

Preamble to the Constitution of the World Health Organization as adopted by the International Health Conference, New York, 19-22 June, 1946; signed on 22 July 1946 by the representatives of 61 States (Official Records of the World Health Organization, no. 2, p. 100) and entered into force on 7 April 1948.

Richard N. Fogoros, M.D. *How Much Exercise is Really Necessary? (2014),* retrieved May 13, 2014 from http://heartdisease.about.com/cs/exercise/a/enoughexercise.htm

ShereenJagtvig, MS *Sun Exposure and Vitamin D(2014)* retrieved on May 13, 2014 from http://nutrition.about.com/od/askyournutritionist/f/sunlight.htm

Wolf R, Wolf D, Rudikoff D, Parish LC. *Nutrition and water: drinking eight glasses of water a day ensures proper skin hydration - myth or reality? ClinDermatol.* 2010;28:380-383.